Mental Health Across Cultures

Mental Health Across Cultures

A PRACTICAL GUIDE FOR HEALTH PROFESSIONALS

JILL BENSON

General Practitioner, Migrant Health Service and Yalata Aboriginal Community
Director, Health in Human Diversity Unit
Discipline of General Practice, University of Adelaide

and

JILL THISTLETHWAITE

Professor in Clinical Education and Research
Director, Institute of Clinical Education
University of Warwick School of Medicine

Foreword by

PROFESSOR MICHAEL KIDD

Professor of General Practice, The University of Sydney
Member at Large, World Organization of Family Doctors (WONCA)
Formerly President, The Royal Australian College of General Practitioners (2002–06)

Radcliffe Publishing
Oxford • New York

Radcliffe Publishing Ltd
18 Marcham Road
Abingdon
Oxon OX14 1AA
United Kingdom

www.radcliffe-oxford.com
Electronic catalogue and worldwide online ordering facility.

British Library Cataloguing in Publication Data

A catalogue record for this book is available from the British Library.

ISBN-13: 978 184619 219 7

Typeset by Pindar NZ, Auckland, New Zealand
Printed and bound by TJI Digital, Padstow, Cornwall, UK

Contents

Foreword

We live in a world where close to 200 000 000 people are living outside their country of origin and where 20 000 000 people are refugees who have fled their own countries because of war, ethnic cleansing or starvation. These extraordinary figures include not just many of the patients attending healthcare facilities, but also many of the people who are providing healthcare services in their adopted countries.

As the different cultures that make up our world become ever more mixed, clinicians face daily challenges in providing care to people of different backgrounds with different beliefs and experiences. Each culture has different styles of communication, problem solving and decision-making. These differences can impact on the presentation and management of mental health concerns.

Jill Benson and Jill Thistlethwaite, the two Jills, are both respected general practitioners and academics with international reputations in mental health and medical education. They have extensive clinical experience working in areas as diverse as refugee health, student health and indigenous health and in urban, rural and remote locations in countries like Australia, Nepal and the United Kingdom.

Together they have authored a brilliant book about mental healthcare across cultures. Cultural challenges can be among the most difficult aspects of clinical medicine. As the two Jills demonstrate, they can also be among the most enjoyable and rewarding.

Every clinician in the world experiences cultural challenges as part of her or his daily work. As we do our best to provide appropriate care to each person who trusts us for their medical care and advice, we are often challenged by cultural barriers. This book provides practical guidance on how to identify, address and overcome these barriers.

The fundamental lesson of this book is that we should listen to our patients and respond appropriately. One of the joys of medicine is that each day our patients confront us with new ways of looking at the world. It is a rare day when a doctor doesn't learn something new about human existence from her or his patients.

The two Jills have interwoven stories from their own patients throughout the book. These are stories of real people who have made an impact on the two authors in their own work as doctors. These stories add great richness to the book's key messages. While some of the stories will make you teary and others will make you laugh, the extraordinary courage of people like Kebedesh, Maggie, Razzaq and Alimamy will inspire you in your own work.

The book discusses different therapies that can be utilised by clinicians and their use in transcultural consultations. The two Jills don't hesitate to tackle the biggest challenges in cross-cultural healthcare delivery; the challenge of prescribing across cultures, the challenge of working through interpreters, the challenge of working alongside traditional healers, the challenge of working with people with different health beliefs to your own. They provide simple advice which can transform these challenges into rewarding aspects of your experience as a clinician.

I commend this book to you and I congratulate the two Jills on their work. This is a book for all healthcare professionals, from students to seasoned clinicians. There are practical lessons in here for us all.

I hope that reading this book helps you to provide better care to all of your own patients, no matter what their and your cultural backgrounds might be.

Michael Kidd
Professor of General Practice, The University of Sydney
Member at Large, World Organization of Family Doctors (WONCA)
President, The Royal Australian College of General Practitioners (2002–06)
August 2008

About the authors

Dr Jill Benson is a general practitioner who is currently Director of the Health in Human Diversity Unit in the Discipline of General Practice, University of Adelaide. She is also a senior medical officer working with refugees at the Migrant Health Service, works at the University Health Practice of the University of Adelaide and with Aboriginal people in the remote community at Yalata. She graduated from Sydney University in 1978, has a Diploma of Child Health from the College of Physicians in London and is a Fellow of the Australian College of Psychological Medicine. She is a member of the Board of STTARS (Survivors of Torture and Trauma Assistance and Rehabilitation Service) and of SAPMEA (South Australian Postgraduate Medical Education Association). In 2005 and 2006 she worked as a locum at a teaching hospital in Dharan in rural Eastern Nepal. She teaches other GPs, students, health professionals and the general public on psychological topics and transcultural health, and sits on various committees, has published papers and presented many times on these topics. Jill is the Australasian representative for the WONCA (World Organization of Family Doctors) Working Party on Mental Health and is an examiner for the AMC (Australian Medical Council). She has presented papers at many conferences and seminars throughout Australia as well as in Lebanon, Florida, Pakistan, Italy, Abu Dhabi, Singapore and Spain.

Professor Jill Thistlethwaite is Professor in Clinical Education and Research, and Director of the Institute of Clinical Education at the University of Warwick School of Medicine from January 2009. She was previously associate professor in medical education in the Faculty of Medicine at the University of Sydney. Jill trained as a general practitioner in the UK and was a full-time principal in general practice in West Yorkshire for 10 years, during which time she became a GP trainer and then course organiser for the Calderdale Vocational

Training Scheme. In 1996, she was appointed senior lecturer in community-based education at the University of Leeds, where she was responsible for the Personal and Professional Development Core Unit of the undergraduate medical programme. She has continued to work part-time as a GP. In 2003, she moved to Australia, first to James Cook University Medical School and then to Sydney. Her interests are consultation skills, interprofessional education and practice, professionalism and women's health. She has published widely in these areas.

Acknowledgements

We would like to thank our patients and colleagues with whom we have interacted during our clinical practice. We have learnt so much from you. In particular we would like to acknowledge those colleagues who contributed to our case studies.

List of boxes, figures and tables

FIGURES

TABLE

SECTION A

Overview and model

Introduction

- About the authors
- Why we wrote this book
- How to use this book

About the authors

We are both general practitioners with diverse career paths and an interest in patients' stories. Our journeys have brought us into contact with people from many cultures and we have worked outside what we would define as our own cultural environments. At the time we were learning to be doctors there was very little in the medical curriculum that focussed on the stories that patients tell and the ways that both the content and the telling are influenced by culture, nature and nurture. We have learnt from experience and mentors. Jill B has extensive experience of working with diverse cultural groups and families, both in Australia and abroad. Her clinical interests include mental health in the primary care setting. She is the Australian representative on the WONCA (World Organization of Family Doctors) Mental Health Working Party. Jill T is now primarily a health professional educator but continues to work as a GP one day a week. She moved from a semi-rural practice in Yorkshire to tropical Australia nearly five years ago. People mainly speak English where she works but language is not the only barrier to understanding and transcultural care.

Our experience

Jill B

Here are stories about two healthcare practices where I'm part of the dominant culture and where others come to consult with me.

Refugees at Migrant Health Service

The Migrant Health Service is a South Australian Health (the state government health service) funded community health service providing specialist primary healthcare services to newly arrived refugees. The multi-disciplinary team includes doctors, nurses, psychologists, social workers and bi-cultural community health workers. I have been working there for the last seven years as a general practitioner seeing patients, writing up protocols, capacity-building, teaching and planning. When I first started working with refugee patients I thought I would mostly be seeing women and that I would be using my skills in cognitive behavioural therapy (CBT). I soon discovered that I needed to rethink my idea of what is a 'negative' thought, of 'normal' reactions to trauma and grief, of the priorities for life and health and of how psychological, social, physical and spiritual aspects of life interact. I learnt quickly that the skills I relied on in my everyday general practice were only a basis on which to build a whole new set of skills. There are many diverse perceptions of health and illness from countries such as the former Yugoslavia, Sudan, Iraq, Afghanistan, Burma, Cambodia, Iran etc that are all very different. I could not possibly learn about every culture in depth but have been able to see patterns of resilience in different groups. Community health workers, interpreters and community leaders are all extremely helpful in filling in many details that I would otherwise have completely missed. The teamwork of the staff continues to be the backbone of any work that is done – both in supporting the patients and in supporting each other.

Learning to be more patient-centred without compromising my own understanding of neuropsychiatry and psychotherapeutic techniques has been a steep learning curve. I needed to learn how to unravel an array of physical symptoms into what might be caused by an unusual infectious disease, what might have a psychological basis and what might need social or community intervention. I have had to modify how I discuss mental illness so as to be more respectful of the social and cultural background of the patients. I have discovered the importance of spirituality and religion for the psychological health of many people from other cultures. This has led me to take what is a courageous step for most doctors and include discussions about a patient's spiritual life as part of their therapy.

To my surprise, I have found that, more than in a general practice setting with people from my own culture, it is the relationship with the therapist that brings the most healing to many of the lives that have been shattered by war, torture and trauma. My race, gender and religion have disappeared in the face of genuine respect, patience and listening skills. I continue to learn.

Students at the University of Adelaide

For the students at the University of Adelaide, the university health service is their local general practice. Many of them are young and are away from their homes in countries such as Malaysia and China for the first time. They are very well educated in their home countries but, because they are studying in English, they often struggle to find the right words, especially when they are distressed and unwell. The pressure to succeed is enormous and the fear of failure often overwhelming. They are vulnerable and sometimes quite lonely. They will often present with symptoms that fit into patterns that I would call anxiety or depression. But these diagnoses may not be acceptable culturally or personally. A different way of working is needed using the physical symptoms with which they present or using 'stress' due to study pressures as a diagnosis. Building up their social networks and stress management skills has been important as well as helping them develop personal resources to deal with their difficulties.

I also come into contact with students who frequent the party scene, use drugs and have multiple sexual partners. This is a lifestyle with which I'm not familiar and I often struggle to maintain a non-judgemental attitude and to treat their illnesses in a respectful way. The use of binge-drinking and drugs to overcome social anxiety disorder, the procrastination that comes with depression and the insecurity that is not remedied by sex are behaviours that I would like to treat as mental health problems. However, many students see these behaviours as normal in people their age and are resistant to my attempts to offer 'help' from the medical profession. I have found that preserving a trusting relationship is of the utmost importance so that if there are consequences of their behaviour, they feel confident that they can come to me for assistance.

The following recounts two practices where I enter into another culture:

Aboriginal community at Yalata

The Yalata Aboriginal community originated when the people who usually settled at Ooldea soak (now Oak Valley) were displaced by the overuse of the water resources by Indian Pacific railway workers, the atomic testing at Maralinga and the opening of the Woomera Rocket Testing Range. They were forcibly removed and resettled in 1952 by the South Australian Government at the newly created Yalata mission about 200km west of Ceduna, on the Far West Coast of South Australia. Yalata is about 290km from the border with Western Australia and about 1180km from Kalgoorlie in Western Australia. Removal from homelands and cultural sites has meant that the Yalata people have been denied their usual way of life and culture and have been forced to live as a single community away from their traditional land. They regard themselves as southern Anangu and speak a dialect of Pitjantjatjara as their first language. The population in Yalata can fluctuate from a core community of around 200 people to up to 500 people depending on the season and on social and cultural issues (e.g. 'sorry business' or funerals, men's business or cultural rites of passage, football matches). About 63% are under 24 years of age and only 6.5% between 45 and 64 years of age, with no-one over the age of 65.[1]

Tullawon Health Service was established in 1984 as an Aboriginal community-controlled health service delivering primary healthcare to the Yalata community. It employs three remote area nurses, four Aboriginal health workers, a mental health nurse and a child health nurse. A doctor from the Royal Flying Doctor Service (RFDS) flies 670km from Port Augusta to run a clinic once a week and to airlift people out if necessary. Specialists and allied health professionals run clinics a few times a year. There is a small community hospital run by the local GPs at Ceduna but there is no public transport and only a few people in the community have drivers' licences. I fly the two and a half hour trip in a small plane from Adelaide two days each month. My job is particularly aimed at medical care for women and children, chronic disease programmes and mental health issues.

Yalata was identified as a community in crisis in 2005 because of the 'family violence, alcohol, substance misuse, unemployment, and low levels of mental and physical health'. The main health and social issues currently seen at Yalata are poor physical health (including ear and skin problems), overcrowding, alcohol, family violence and mental health issues. The average life expectancy is 43.3 years, despite the decline in alcohol consumption and petrol sniffing.[1]

Working in a remote Aboriginal community is very different to working in an urban general practice. The doctor is a small part of a team that includes the remote area nurses, Aboriginal health workers, mental health workers, the Royal Flying Doctor Service (RFDS), Ngankaris (traditional healers), community elders, teachers, police, shopkeepers and many other people. The nurses screen, diagnose, prescribe, manage and organise retrievals by the RFDS. As a doctor who flies in and flies out for only a few days each month, I'm mainly acting as a consultant and a support, helping co-ordinate chronic disease programmes as well as doing one-on-one consultations. Other health professionals such as dentists, audiologists, ophthalmologists and psychiatrists fly in a few times a year. Consultations are held in the health service facility, in the school, under a tree, in the home – wherever the patient happens to be. There is no on-site pathology or radiology, and medicine relies very much on clinical and relationship skills. If patients need specialist consultations, X-rays or admission to hospital they need to be flown out by the RFDS, be taken 200km to Ceduna by the nurse or convince someone who can drive to take them to Ceduna, 670km to Port Augusta or 970km to Adelaide. Nothing happens unless there is a good relationship with the patient, with the community and with the other staff.

On my first visit to the community I was to be interviewed by some of the women who had asked for a woman doctor to be employed in the area. We all sat around in a room and I waited for someone to ask me a question. None came. They actually had all the information they needed about me from other Aboriginal women I had worked with who had 'vouched' for me. I talked about some of the other doctors and nurses I knew who had worked in the community and who had sent their regards to the local people. Everyone found this much more interesting than a formal interview.

I was concerned that I did not have a 'mentor', someone who could tell me if I was making cultural mistakes and help me negotiate cross-cultural problems. In my previous practice my mentor was a wonderful elder woman who would answer all my bumbling questions with patience and good humour. I also knew that if I unconsciously did anything culturally inappropriate that she would hear about it and would be at my doorstep to tell me. My mentors at Yalata are the Aboriginal health workers. They are very experienced and act as 'brokers' with the community as well as their usual health worker roles.

Nepalese people at BPKoirala Institute of Health Sciences (BPKIHS) in Dharan in Eastern Nepal

Nepal, with a population of about 25 million people, is one of the poorest countries in the world. They are mostly farmers living in rural areas but are of several ethnic groups and religions.[2] Life expectancy is about 60 years and 40% of the population is under the age of 15.[3] Over the last ten years there have been frequent natural disasters and political conflicts that have disrupted much of the fragile health system. Infectious diseases, malnutrition, infant and maternal mortality and public health issues are the main health issues in the country and take priority over mental health in both government and non-government organisation (NGO) programmes.[4] There are 18 outpatient mental health facilities in the country, three day-treatment facilities, 17 community-based psychiatric inpatient units and one mental hospital. The majority of patients are treated in outpatient facilities and most psychiatric services operate out of major cities.[5]

In Nepal there are only 40 psychiatrists and 60 general practitioners in the entire country. Australia, with a similar population, has about 3000 psychiatrists and about 20 000 GPs.[5] The stigma that is associated with mental health issues 'rubs off' on the health professionals who work with those who are mentally ill from both the medical as well as the general community. Psychiatrists and psychologists will sometimes be ostracised by their colleagues and families for choosing mental health as a career.[6,7]

Mental disorders account for 11.1% of the total burden of disease in some developing countries.[8] Factors such as poverty, low education levels, conflict, disasters and gender disadvantage increase the risk of mental disorders in developing countries above those in developed countries.[8] Bad fortune, life stresses, social conflict and evil spirits may be blamed for mental health problems, and traditional and religious therapies are mostly used for treatment. There is limited 'mental health literacy' or 'mental health promotion' so mental illness is rarely seen as a medical problem. Patients are more likely to present with somatic symptoms or in a 'trance' from evil spirits than with psychological symptoms that would lead to a diagnosis of anxiety or depression.

The BPKIHS is a university that was established in 1993 at the old British Ghurkha camp at Ghopa on the outskirts of Dharan, a town of 100 000. It is about 13 hours east of Kathmandu and serves the east of Nepal. It is funded through collaboration between the Nepali and Indian governments. There is a 700-bed teaching hospital that provides tertiary-level healthcare for about two million people, with a special concern for the poor. Medical care is not free for most patients, but 10% of the budget is used for the care of those who have run out of money. This can happen quite quickly in intensive care, and deters many poor people from coming to the hospital at all. There are about 850 medical, dental, nursing and public health students and about 5000 people living in the university/hospital complex.

Up to 400 people start to arrive from dawn each day to attend General Outpatients. Some have walked three days to get there and some have camped overnight with their family and animals in the hospital car park. Each patient, no matter what their age or illness, has a 'patient party' who will run and buy medication, take blood specimens to the laboratory, take an X-ray to the radiology department for reporting etc, but will also take an active part in the consultation, discussing symptoms, explaining what the doctor or the patient has said in more detail and taking part in any decision-making. Sometimes the 'patient party' is a spouse or a relative, but sometimes it is a friend or a group of elders from the village. They sit or stand behind the patient throughout the consultation.

There are five consulting rooms, each with one desk in the middle piled with paperwork, a bed at each end, one with a tattered screen, and a small collection of equipment such as speculums, a sphygmomanometer and a tendon hammer. Two or three doctors work in each room, on opposite sides of the desk. Up to 15 people can be crammed into an ordinary-sized consulting room at any one time, discussing the intimate details of their health. Confidentiality is difficult but the lack of it does not seem to worry the Nepalese people.

The Emergency Department is a similar mixture of patients, friends, relatives and onlookers milling around a very small area with limited equipment and the maximum number of beds and mattresses. Death is frequent in a country where infectious diseases such as malaria, TB, typhoid and Japanese encephalitis are common and difficult to treat because of lack of medication, poverty, distance and malnutrition. Suicide by hanging or organophosphate poisoning occurs all too often and people are occasionally brought in after being shot or wounded in the local 'civil war'.

I have been to BPKIHS twice, for a month each time, to work with other Australian doctors in the Department of Family Medicine and to do some teaching in the Department of Psychiatry. I plan to go for a month each year but the politics have made this difficult in recent times. On my first visit to Nepal I 'did my best' but was often very distressed by the feeling of loneliness and hopelessness of the situation. I spent a lot of time preparing myself for my second visit, took two other doctors with me, laughed more, had more teaching resources and paced myself better. I did not know much more clinically but had learnt new ways of teaching the students, new ways of accessing psychological issues in a culture where mental health is a virtually unknown area and new ways of setting boundaries and caring for myself.

Our experience

Jill T

As a GP registrar and subsequently a GP in a semi-rural area of Yorkshire, England, I would have thought I was very much a part of the culture of the countryside. However, with the naivety of youth, doctors often feel they know a lot and have all the skills to make a difference. Then we encounter the 85-year-old lady who has never travelled further than the big town five miles away, or the travellers who want treatment for scabies but do not want their children vaccinated. As a young doctor I interacted with couples whose marriages were coming apart due to the stress of infertility, parents with very sick children, people who could not afford to pay for their prescriptions – all very different life stresses to those I had known. The empathic GP learns to listen and not jump to conclusions. When I moved to Australia I thought the culture would be a little different but not too strange – English-speaking but warmer. But each health system is a new culture to be navigated through – the complexities and bureaucracy must be a nightmare for those who do not have the language skills. It is funny what you miss of your own country and the homesickness that creeps up now and then. The networks I had built up over 16 years in one practice, the knowledge of which doctors to refer to, how to access allied health professionals and 'my patients' were all lost to me half a world away.

Listening is even more important with the patient population I interact with at the health centre at the University of Sydney. The patients are predominantly under 30 years of age. They consult about sexual health, for contraception, for university-related stress and mental health problems. Many of the students are from overseas with English as a second or even third or fourth language. I also need to be able to ask the right questions. Doctors are seen as influential people by some of the overseas students – we should know what is wrong! Thinking of the words to discuss female problems is difficult when the person sitting across from me does not know what a smear test is, or an internal examination or a vaginal discharge. It takes two, three or more consultations to gain someone's trust enough to move on past the biomedical-type history to the person's story. I haven't got the mental images to go with the life they have left behind. I can understand a little of the culture shock but not the day-to-day difficulties of living in a very strange land where there is often impatience with poor language skills and discrimination.

Being seen as an educator I have been asked to facilitate cultural diversity workshops and help other health professionals learn about cultural safety. This would not be possible without the cultural mentors I have met and their generosity in helping me with my culture shock. The communication and consultation skills I help learners develop are constantly being refined personally as I learn from my interactions with patients and other health professionals.

Doctors are predominantly being asked to work within an evidence-based framework. However, this can be difficult. Female students from the USA are used to having a full gynaecological examination and cervical (pap) smear every year. In Australia the recommended interval is two years and in the UK smears are taken every three to five years depending on age. How does one explain this to a patient? A woman who has been told it is imperative to be screened every year is now advised this is unnecessary. This is a simple example of different expectations and it is easy to understand how patients become confused and suspicious, especially when health professionals do not interact with them in the same way in every country.

Personal reflection on 'culture shock'

I moved from one English-speaking country (UK) to another (Australia) at the other end of the world. We appeared to share a similar cultural heritage. While I had few problems with communication (the language was mainly the same) the biggest shock was the difference in the health system. Having worked within the British National Health Service I was unused to charging patients and was unclear as to the fees they would face when I prescribed, requested investigations or arranged referrals. When discussing options with patients for the management of mental health problems, I often found that patients factored into their decision the cost implications. Taking an antidepressant could be cheaper than seeing a psychologist. Consultations were much more anxious affairs for me as I tried to cope with unfamiliar drug names, lack of allied health professionals under the same roof, which meant that interprofessional discussions and advice were more difficult to obtain, and the hierarchy of charges. I could empathise with the much more difficult situation of new doctors who also had language and cultural barriers; and the frustration of patients wanting to engage with their health provider but feeling that they were misunderstood.

Why we wrote this book

The World Health Organization has predicted that by the year 2020 depression will be the second leading cause of disability-adjusted life years (DALYs) for all ages and sexes. It is already one of the most common causes of disability in the world.[9] The increase in depression is most likely a multifactorial phenomenon due to biological (e.g. longevity, chronic diseases, stress), psychological (e.g. loss of meaning, learned helplessness, loneliness) and sociocultural and environmental (e.g. role confusion, urbanisation, cultural disintegration) causes.[10] It is imperative that health professionals improve their skills in dealing with depression, not only within their usual cultural milieu, but so as to properly understand, assess and treat depression in an increasingly multicultural world.

Health professionals, wherever they work, will interact with patients from a different culture to their own. While learning from and reflection on experience is helpful, too often we can make disastrous mistakes along the way – alienating patients, misunderstanding cues and stories, offering the wrong management plan at the worse time or feeling hopeless when we have no idea what is wrong with the patient or how to help them. Health professionals want to work better, to provide optimum patient care and to do this in a multicultural society. This book is aimed at those professionals who want to know more about transcultural consultations and how to improve communication.

It is written from an evidence-based point of view but it is also written from experience, and scattered throughout the text are case studies to illustrate points and bring the human being back into the equation.

This book is not just about working in mental health in a different country. Psychological health permeates every field of health and whether you are a neurosurgeon or a nurse assistant, skills in dealing with mental health across cultures are of the utmost importance. Culture is not just about what country we come from or who our parents were. It also includes differences in gender, spiritual beliefs, sexual orientation, lifestyle, beliefs, age, social status or perceived economic worth.[11] We may have more in common with many of the other middle-aged, highly-educated doctors in remote Nepal than we do with some of the young students we see at an Australian university health practice. Wherever we work, whoever we are, we are working across cultures, often without realising it. The first step is to become conscious of this fact. The next step is to read this book.

How to use this book

Note: We describe interactions as occurring with patients, as we are both doctors. However, we recognise that other health professionals would be more comfortable with nomenclature such as clients, consumers or service users. Ultimately, it should really be the person seeking advice or help who decides on terminology. We also use personal pronouns such as he/she and his/her to help the flow of the text; these are not meant to be exclusive.

Section A: The first section is an overview of a model for working in mental health across cultures. This can be used as personal preparation for health professionals who are working across cultures or as a teaching tool for use with health professionals who are travelling to another culture (such as overseas aide workers) or health professionals who have moved to a new country (such as international medical graduates).

Section B: This section outlines some practical ways of using psychotherapy skills across cultures and new concepts such as resilience and spirituality that may need to be consolidated.

Section C: This section broadens some of the concepts from the previous two sections and explores some of the evidence base for cross-cultural mental health in practice and for teaching purposes.

REFERENCES

1 Family and Community Services (FaCS). Yalata multi purpose community centre to improve family well being and reduce family violence. Attorney-General's Department, Canberra; 2005.

2 Regmi S, Pokharel A, Ojha S, *et al.* Nepal mental health country profile. *Int Rev Psychiatry.* 2004; **16**: 142–9.

3 World Health Organization, Ministry of Health and Population of Nepal. *WHO-AIMS Report on Mental Health System in Nepal.* Kathmandu, Nepal; 2006.

4 Vijayakumar L, Pirkis J, Whiteford H. Suicide in developing countries (3): prevention efforts. *Crisis.* 2005; **26**: 120–4.

5 Jacob K, Sharan P, Mirza I, *et al.* Mental health systems in countries: where are we now? *Lancet.* 2007; **370**: 1061–77.

6 Arboleda-Florez J. Considerations on the stigma of mental illness. *Can J Psychiatry.* 2003; **48**: 645–50.

7 Shakya R. Personal communication. Dharan, Nepal; 2008.

8 Patel V. Mental health in low- and middle-income countries. *Br Med Bull.* 2007; **81–82**: 81–96.

9 World Health Organization. *Depression.* 2008. Available at: www.who.int/mental_health/management/depression/definition/en/ (accessed April 2008).

10 Marsella A, Kaplan A, Suarez E. Cultural considerations for understanding, assessing, and treating depressive experience and disorder. In: Reinecke M, Davison M, editors. *Comparative Treatments of Depression.* New York: Springer Series on Comparative Treatments for Psychological Disorders; 2002. pp. 47–78.

11 Medical Council of New Zealand. *Statement on Cultural Competence.* 2006. Available at: www.mcnz.org.nz/portals/0/guidance/cultural%20competence.pdf (accessed April 2007).

Model for working in mental health across cultures

This chapter explores the following model:

BOX 2.1 MODEL FOR WORKING IN MENTAL HEALTH ACROSS CULTURES (ADAPTED FROM VICARY AND BISHOP)[1]

1 Self-reflection on cultural context
2 Networking and mentoring
   Cultural mentors
3 Review of psychotherapy skills
4 Management team
5 Hearing the patient's story
   Cultural Awareness Tool
6 Potential barriers
7 Choosing appropriate therapeutic options
8 Follow-up of the patient
9 Boundaries and self-care
10 Evaluation of the process

We discuss and expand on this model for working in transcultural mental health. Each of the 10 parts begins with an overview in bullet points and continues with a short explanation. The model represents important aspects and stages of working in consultations across cultures. A more detailed explanation is provided in chapters of Section B and C.

1 SELF-REFLECTION ON CULTURAL CONTEXT

➤ In each culture there are different communication styles, attitudes toward conflict, approaches to completing tasks, notions of time, decision-making styles, attitudes toward disclosure and approaches to knowledge and health.

➤ Only a small percentage of motives, beliefs and reactions are conscious.

➤ The 'ethnocentrism' of the mental health professional needs to be conscious in order to recognise properly the cultural beliefs and expectations of the patient.

➤ This is more important in cross-cultural consultations with the potential for miscommunication and lack of understanding.

➤ Reflection on the cultural context and its effects on interactions are important.

The majority of health professionals start medicine wanting to contribute, save lives, help people and have social importance and/or a good job with a stable income. However, not all such motives and reactions are likely to be conscious.[2] Health professionals are likely to be conscientious and perfectionists, have a marked sense of responsibility, a need for control and for people-pleasing, be chronically self-doubting and able to delay gratification, but they also have a sense of entitlement to a level of prestige and respect for their hard work or role in society. Some may be unconsciously attempting to give patients all the love and care they didn't receive as children. Health professionals are likely to struggle with their own limitations, and may feel depressed or a failure when not every patient is able to be cured or saved.[3] This outcome is likely to be even more pronounced in cross-cultural consultations with the potential for miscommunication and lack of understanding. Because of their perfectionist nature, many health professionals do not deal well with uncertainty or lack of success. They may become defensive or guilty or even blame patients if their problems are not getting better. Or they may refer the patient on to someone else who they think might be able to solve the problem, without stopping to think that the patient will have to start their difficult story all over again.

In each culture there are different communication styles, attitudes toward conflict, approaches to completing tasks, notions of time, decision-making styles, attitudes toward disclosure and approaches to knowledge.[4] Usually, cultural style and expectations are unconscious, both in the individual and tacitly within the wider society. For example, the use of the term culturally and linguistically diverse (CALD) applied to a person implies that everyone else is diverse but 'us'. This is a curious term in a country like Australia where

24% of the population is born overseas[5] and in the UK with its long history of immigration. 'Ethnocentrism' refers to this tendency for each person to perceive reality from the vantage point of their own cultural experience.[6]

Whether people's patterns of behaviour, thinking and feeling are being noticed at all and, if so, whether they are described in moral, psychosocial or medical terms is influenced by local culture and society and usually varies over time.[7] The power of Western psychiatric diagnoses does not mean that they are accurate, merely that they are dominant, because of the current economic, political, academic and military dominance of the West.[6] Whether a health professional is working from the stance of the Western dominant culture or not, it is always essential to explore the expectations of the individual patient and to aim the therapy towards a mutually acceptable goal.

It is important for health professionals not to stereotype patients into cultures or subgroups, even those who are from the same background as themselves. For instance, doctors are likely to have a very different 'culture' to other people who have grown up in the same region because of their education, wealth, lifestyle and social position. They may lose sight of what 'ordinary' people do in their lives and unconsciously make value judgements based on their own ethnocentric views.

Every society has a 'culture' of mental health that has been built up over many decades. Even within the last 30 years, for example, schizophrenia has been viewed as a spiritual problem, a family problem, a genetic problem or a drug-related problem. History shows that the definition of 'normal' also changes over time, being affected by biomedical research, society's evolution, philosophy and governments. This will affect the definitions of mental illness, deviance, eccentricity or even 'alternative'. In the field of mental health, clinicians are more susceptible to misdiagnosis through value judgements because there is no objective test of normality but rather a sequence of symptoms and signs, perhaps backed up by health questionnaires, which lead to labelling.

Despite being criticised regularly for its Western viewpoint of mental illness, the *Diagnostic and Statistical Manual of Mental Disorders* (the DSM-IV) of the American Psychiatric Association states that 'diagnostic assessment can be especially challenging when a clinician from one ethnic or cultural group uses the DSM-IV. A clinician who is unfamiliar with the nuances of an individual's cultural frame of reference may incorrectly judge as psychopathology those normal variations in behaviour, belief, or experience that are particular to the individual's culture'.[8] Somatoform disorders, factitious disorder, abnormal grief reaction and abnormal illness behaviour are just some of the diagnoses patients from a different culture may be given inappropriately in a Western framework. To make a diagnosis of mental illness, the patient's symptoms must be deemed abnormal within their own culture and be interfering with their ability to live a normal life as defined by themselves and/or by their community or culture.

The life experiences of patients and health professionals will influence how the two inter-relate. Refugees, overseas students and migrants into developed countries may have physical and psychological problems very different to those of patients their health professionals usually treat. Likewise, health professionals trained within different cultures and themselves the victims of hardship and discrimination may have difficulty accepting that certain mental health problems of patients, who appear to have no major life traumas, are worthy of medical consideration. We must also remember that spirituality pervades every aspect of the lives of people from most indigenous cultures and cannot be differentiated from either their physical or mental well-being.[9]

2 NETWORKING AND MENTORING

➤ Communication and developing an understanding of the 'cultural reality' of a community.
➤ Building relationships and networks with people who can help the health professional research the community's beliefs and traditions.
➤ The need to develop trust, skills and knowledge to dispel the myths and stereotypes of both patients and practitioner.
➤ The role of cultural mentors.

Working across cultures is not just about evidence-based practice. Communication and developing an understanding of the 'cultural reality' of a community are essential if the health professional is going to be working within that culture or with people from specific cultural groups long-term. This means building relationships and networks with people who can help the health professional research the community's beliefs and traditions. This may be through community health workers, local elders, teachers or even local shopkeepers. Some of the relationships may be professional and the issue of cultural awareness will need to be discussed as part of that relationship. Others may be informal or even social. 'Immersion' in the community is probably the most helpful way of learning about a culture, as the subtle nuances of social taboos and accomplishments are likely to be unconscious.[10] It may be that the health professional needs to become involved in another aspect of community life such as the arts or sport. However, care must be taken to ensure that boundary issues and support are properly addressed (*see* step 9).

An attitude of curiosity and respect will be needed to guide this quest so that a non-judgemental and safe environment is generated from the beginning.[11] This will usually take patience and perseverance and it may take years to develop the trust, skills and knowledge to dispel the myths and stereotypes of both patients and professionals.[12] If the health professional approaches this task with humility and good will, the community is more than likely to be helpful and forgiving of mistakes.

Cultural mentors

A cultural mentor or consultant is a 'teacher, counselor, parent, historian, politician, anthropologist and psychologist'.[13] A cultural mentor can interpret and 'broker' so that the health professional can learn what rules and conventions apply and the different ways in which people decide what is important, how activities are allocated, how decisions are made, how respect is shown and how time is observed.[14] 'Vouching' by a senior and respected person from the community means that other people are likely to be more confident about talking to someone from a different culture.[1] Vouching involves the endorsement of a person or a service to others because they have been happy with the assistance they have been given and with the relationship with the health professional.

Communication skills might be learnt from discussions with the cultural mentors such as the meaning of eye contact or body language. In some cultures it is disrespectful to look people in the face or in the eyes and looking away is a sign of respect. In others it is impolite to answer a question in the negative and so it will be difficult to get a history if direct questions with yes/no answers are asked. Many cultures have gender taboos about what can be discussed with a member of the opposite sex and especially about whether someone can be examined. Similarly, there may be problems if the practitioner is younger than the patient. Some cultures have taboos about saying certain names or talking to certain members of their own or another family group. For every culture there will be subtle meanings and taboos which are likely to get in the way of easy communication. A health professional will never be able to learn all of these and so needs to constantly be aware of problems that may arise and have access to a cultural mentor with which to discuss these.

3 REVIEW OF PSYCHOTHERAPY SKILLS

➤ Consulting and counselling skills will need to be reviewed and may need modification to work successfully across cultures.
➤ Family therapy and group therapy skills may need to be learnt.

➤ Therapy should be holistic, using traditional, spiritual, psychosocial and biomedical models to explain and treat mental illness.

➤ Mental health problems may manifest spiritually and culturally and therefore may only be resolved in this manner.

➤ Culture-bound illnesses may conform to DSM-IV criteria but have a different cause and therefore require a more appropriate and varied treatment regime.

➤ Culture-bound syndromes are recurrent, cultural-specific patterns of abnormal behaviour and/or troubling experience that do not necessarily conform with a specific DSM-IV diagnosis.[8]

The therapeutic skills that equip a health professional to work successfully in a Western environment are not necessarily going to be useful in working across cultures. Consulting and counselling skills will need to be reviewed and may need modification. Some skills might be learnt through trial and error, such as the inappropriateness of reflective feedback, which might be seen as inter-ruption in some cultures, or the direct line of questioning, which may be seen as confrontational or rude.[10]

There must be 'an opportunity within the assessment process to explore the extent to which the particular mental health issue is symptomatic of the individual's underlying cultural and/or spiritual issues. Often, it is the case that mental health problems will manifest themselves spiritually and culturally and therefore can often only be resolved in this manner.'[12] Serious illness is often attributed to external forces or reasons, for example people may attribute illness to some external wrongdoing, breaching of taboos or cultural responsibility. Culture-bound illnesses may conform to DSM-IV criteria but have a different cause and therefore require a more appropriate and varied treatment regime. For example, in Australian Aboriginal culture 'longing for, crying for, or being sick for country' follows the same symptom base as depression. However, the cause is the individual's removal from their country, place of dreaming or spirit for extended periods of time. The resolution involves a combination of traditional treatment with Westernised forms of psychotherapy.[12] Aboriginal people may also have a more fatalistic view of depression as a personal characteristic of the individual concerned, stating 'that's just the way he is'.[12] This means that depression may go unnoticed and even traditional methods of interpretation and healing may not be activated.

Being well in the world view of many cultures incorporates cultural and spiritual elements as well as physical and mental aspects of health. Other factors that may be seen to have an impact on a person's wellness include employment status, substance abuse, family violence, dispossession, cultural identity and housing and financial problems.[12,15] Whatever it is that the patient presents as the main problem needs to be the focus for the health professional. A Western-style therapy concentrating on psychological symptoms is not going to succeed if the patient's presenting problem is physical, social, spiritual or cultural.

As well as skills such as cognitive behavioural therapy (CBT), the health professional will need to know how to use more patient-focussed therapies such as narrative therapy, or at least refer to an appropriate professional who can. They will need to be familiar with a style of questioning such as that of the Cultural Awareness Tool (see below) that allows a patient to discuss the priorities in his or her own life and mental health rather than the priorities expected by the health professional. Group therapy and family therapy are distinct skills that may need to be learnt by health professionals if they are working in a culture where consultations are mostly with a family rather than an individual. Even expertise in the use of interpreters should not be taken for granted, especially when discussing psychological health, and may need to be enhanced.

4 MANAGEMENT TEAM

➤ The team includes all health and social care professionals, plus traditional healers involved in working with the patient, the family and the community as appropriate.
➤ It is important to know how patients access the GP or other health professional.
➤ In collectivist communities the health professional should ask the patient who should be involved in the consultation and where it should be held.
➤ Traditional healers could play a role in:
  — managing stress-related disorders
  — becoming active case-finders
  — facilitating referrals
  — providing counselling, monitoring and follow-up care
  — working with the health professional when mental illness is linked to breaches of forbidden and sacred relationships, which could be addressed effectively only within protocols laid down in the culture.

It is important to know how patients come to be seeing the GP or health professional. This will help build up an idea of what their expectations might be. If referrals are made through the community health worker, traditional healer, elder or another health professional in the community, the GP will already have been 'vouched' for as someone to be trusted.

In more collectivist communities it is important for the therapist to ask the patient who should be involved in the consultation and where the consultation should be held (especially if it involves children). Issues such as seating arrangements, which are important in family and group therapy, will also need to be discussed with the other people who attend the consultation. Who does most of the talking, who takes responsibility for treatment and follow-up, who organises investigations etc – in fact, most of the issues that a practitioner might usually discuss with an individual – may need to be discussed with the family and management team as well. The patients and family need to be part of the decision-making about referrals to other health professionals who may not have the same cross-cultural skills as the health professional they have originally chosen, or there may be taboos such as gender that will need to be taken into account.

Traditional healers, complementary therapists and religious leaders provide up to 80% of the care received by the mentally ill throughout the world.[16,17] Some patients may believe in the curative power of non-medical interventions, such as God or traditional folk medicine and healers, which precludes the use of medication.[18] Acknowledging and respecting the part that traditional healers, elders and alternative health practitioners play in the mental health of the community is problematic for many health professionals.

Setting up a working relationship with traditional healers is difficult because of the stereotypes that both professions have about each other. The suggestion to do so may come from the patients themselves as a trusting relationship develops with the health professional. It will only be when all parties are in agreement that a working relationship can develop between the traditional healer and the health professional. For Western health professionals who are working in more traditional communities, the cultural mentor may be able to liaise between the two.

Traditional healers can play an increased role in managing stress-related disorders. They can be active case finders, and can facilitate referral and provide counselling, monitoring and follow-up care.[19] Mental ill health is sometimes linked to breaches of forbidden and sacred relationships, which could be addressed effectively only within protocols laid down in the culture. Doctors and traditional healers can work together to help address many such mental health problems.

In many Western medical practices there is now more cooperation between complementary therapists and more conventional medicine. Referrals for acupuncture, hypnotherapy, naturopathy or therapeutic massage are becoming more and more common. The enormous budget spent on vitamins each year in Western countries, the fact that many health funds in countries like Australia are now subsidising visits to chiropractors, homeopaths and reflexologists, and that British health professionals learn acupuncture skills bears witness to the general acceptance by the community of what have previously been seen as alternative healing techniques. Doctors need to take note that some of the reasons people prefer to go to alternative therapists are because they spend more time building a relationship with the patient and are better listeners. The movement of medicine in many Western countries towards large group practices, where doctors do not have the time or interest in establishing a good relationship with patients or families, is only likely to exacerbate this problem. It is important that Western practitioners acknowledge that healing is not just from the use of 'left brain' techniques such as talking therapies, but also from the 'right brain' practices of many alternative therapies, including the relationship between patient and practitioner.

5 HEARING THE PATIENT'S STORY

➤ The patient's story must always be seen in the context of the culture of origin as well as the present culture.
➤ It is important to find a balance between confidentiality and involving the patient, family and community.
➤ An experienced interpreter will be needed if the patient and health professional speak different languages because:
  — the patient's first language will be the one with which they have access to dreams, childhood memories, world view and many deeply held cultural beliefs
  — the patient may find it difficult to find words to explain feelings in a second language in a stressful situation.

Clarifying the context of a patient's demographics when working in mental health across cultures will involve more than the usual age, gender, language, occupation, co-morbidities and family history. It may also involve other aspects such as culture of origin, dialect, religion, education, length of time in the new country, history of the journey to the new country, who is left behind, current social supports, previous occupation, history of torture and trauma, lifestyle and who 'grew up' the patient (i.e. who was their main primary caregiver as a child). The most important part of the history-taking, however, will be the narrative as presented by the patient, and the respectful and careful listening by the therapist. Many of the questions above will be answered with this strategy without direct questions being asked.

There are different cultural concepts that will influence the way a patient presents their story to a health professional. The first is the ethnocentrism of the patient – their natural tendency to view reality from their own cultural experience and perspective. Of course, there will be their culture – the shared learned meanings and behaviours that are transmitted from within a social context and which are represented both externally (e.g. roles) and internally (e.g. values, beliefs). But it is also important to take into account the new ethnocultural identity of the patient who has moved to another culture. This refers to the 'extent to which an individual endorses and manifests the cultural traditions and practices of a particular group'.[20] Some people will resolutely maintain their cultural traditions, some will become acculturated and some will develop a third culture by 'creolisation' that blends both traditions.[21,22] This last point involves people selecting elements of both their culture of origin and of the receiving culture to form a sort of hybrid culture.

History and information can be gathered from the patient, the family, the referrer or the cultural mentor. For those who come from a collectivist culture, the whole history may come from the family or close community members. In many cultures all issues of importance are usually discussed collectively, even when this is about the health of an adult.[23] For many patients shame will play a big part in what they are prepared to share with a 'stranger' and there will need to be a cultural intermediary such as a community health worker involved. It is important to find a balance between confidentiality and involving the patient, family and community.[24] This will need to be guided by the patient and the cultural mentor as appropriate.

Mental health and mental illness may not be familiar concepts in many cultures. Therefore, asking if the patient has or has had mental health problems may not elicit a response. Symptoms of mental health problems may only be conceived in physical terms because there are no words for psychological illness in the language, because that is how the people understand their illness or because this is the only way they can communicate how they're feeling. How someone copes within a community, their resilience and where the line is between 'normal' and 'abnormal' is both individual and societal.[11]

Cultural Awareness Tool

Symptoms of mental health problems may only be conceived in physical terms because:

➤ there are no words for psychological illness in the language
➤ that is how the people understand their illness
➤ this is the only way patients can communicate how they're feeling.

The Cultural Awareness Tool[25] (Box 2.2) is based on a series of questions developed by Arthur Kleinman in 1978[26] that acknowledge that the patient is the expert on his or her own life and culture.[27] A patient's 'degree of distress, illness behaviour, pattern of help-seeking and compliance or non-compliance with recommended treatment become understandable in the light of the way in which he or she answers each of these questions'.[28]

BOX 2.2 CULTURAL AWARENESS TOOL

What do you think caused your problem?

Why do you think it started when it did?

What do you think illness does to you?

What are the chief problems it has caused for you?

How severe is your illness?

What do you most fear about it?

What kind of treatment/help do you think you should receive?

Within your own culture how would your illness be treated?

How are your family and community helping you?

What have you been doing so far?

What are the most important results you hope to get from treatment?

When would you like to come back?

The use of these questions can assist health professionals in discussing cultural problems and exploring the aetiology, expectations and possible solutions without being fully aware of the patient's cultural background or compromising their beliefs.[26] The questions reflect the usual movement of a consultation through symptoms, past history, assessment of severity, safety issues, treatment, safety net and so on. With experience in different cultural settings, the style of questioning can be refined and rendered more specific for that culture. They can also become more 'embedded' as part of a generalised conversational flow.[26] Gathering information through a normal conversation rather than through questioning is less threatening to patients and allows them the opportunity to acknowledge symptoms that may otherwise be difficult for them to express verbally.[29]

BOX 2.3 CASE STUDY 1 (SIMON'S STORY FEATURING USE OF THE CULTURAL AWARENESS TOOL)

Simon, a recently arrived refugee from Sudan, presented to the doctor complaining of stomach pain. The doctor diagnosed gastro-oesophageal reflux and gave him some medication.

He presented again three weeks later with the same problem. The doctor decided to use the Cultural Awareness Tool.

What do you think caused your problem?
I think I have a worm in my stomach that is causing this problem. It has been there a long time, since I was in Africa.

Why do you think it started when it did?
It started in 1997 when the war came to our village. My parents and my two brothers were killed. I escaped with my wife and our young child. We had to run a very long way and we were very hungry. We drank bad water at that time and I think this is when the worm started to take hold of me.

What do you think this illness does to you?
As well as giving me stomach pain this worm has made me lose my appetite, has made me tired, it stops me sleeping, gives me headaches and makes me irritable all the time.

What are the chief problems it has caused for you?
Because I am not sleeping and am so irritable I can't go to school, I yell at my wife and children and I'm not seeing my friends.

How severe is your illness?
It is very severe this worm. I'm afraid it will take all the energy from me and I may even die.

What do you most fear about it?
I'm afraid that it may kill me but also that my wife may leave me and take the children.

What kind of treatment/help do you think you should receive?
I think I should receive some strong worm treatment and also be given something that will give me my energy back and help my brain to think normally again.

Within your own culture, how would your illness be treated?
When I was in Africa and I first noticed this worm, I went to see the traditional healer. He gave me some medicine and asked me to come back every two

weeks to talk about my condition and receive more medicine. I improved with this medicine but I don't think you can get it here.

How are your family and community helping you?
I have not told anyone in the community that I have this worm. I'm ashamed that I'm yelling at my wife and children and that I'm so irritable. My wife is kind and says that this is the worm causing the problem and that I am really a good man. She is the one who has told me to come and see you again.

What have you been doing so far?
I have been hiding in my room a great deal as I don't want to go out. Sometimes I sing to myself to try to distract myself from the problems the worm is causing me. Sometimes early in the morning I go for long walks while everyone else is still asleep. I have taken some worm medicine from the chemist and I've taken the medicine that you have given me but it hasn't helped.

What are the most important results you hope to get from treatment?
I'm hoping that my stomach pain and headaches will get better and that I will have more energy. But I'm also hoping that I can laugh with my children again, talk happily with my wife, go back to school, and sing and play football with my friends.

When would you like to come back?
I think you should give me some medicine and I should come back regularly to be sure the medicine is working.

On this occasion the doctor diagnosed Simon with depression. She decided to test his stools for worms but also discussed how depression can cause fatigue, irritability and physical symptoms. Simon agreed to try some antidepressants. The doctor also helped Simon to focus on his positive attributes – his love for his family and their love for him; his ability to find activities like singing and walking to distract him from his depression; and his courage and strength in managing to bring his family to safety in the face of overwhelming danger and hardship. She was only able to discover all these attributes because she asked questions such as those above. The usual blunt, disease-focussed line of questioning would not have revealed the true nature of Simon's condition.

Simon's stools revealed *Giardia lamblia*, for which he was given medication, and after six sessions of narrative therapy and six months of antidepressants he announced that he was well and stopped further treatment.

6 POTENTIAL BARRIERS

➤ Patient factors.

➤ Clinician factors.

➤ Healthcare system factors.

➤ Societal and environmental factors.

Barriers will need to be addressed from the outset if a good therapeutic relationship is to be established.

Patient factors

Patients progress through several stages before seeking treatment: experiencing symptoms, evaluating the severity and consequences of symptoms, assessing whether treatment is required, assessing the feasibility of and options for treatment, deciding whether to seek treatment and accessing care.[30] Barriers can appear at any of these stages, especially if the patient's understanding of psychological symptomatology is limited or culturally unacceptable. Most patients do not recognise their symptoms as depression and focus on the somatic complaints that are part of the illness such as gastrointestinal problems, fatigability, headaches, pain and sleep problems.[31] It is up to the health professional to be aware that these symptoms may have an underlying cause that is psychological. People who actually present with psychological complaints are more likely to be recognised than those who somatise, normalise or minimise their symptoms.[32]

Clinician factors

The main barriers relating to the clinician are: poor education about psychopharmacology and psychotherapy for depression, limited training in interpersonal skills to manage emotional distress, avoidance of addressing mental health problems, inadequate time to evaluate and treat depression, failure to consider psychotherapeutic approaches, fear of alienating patients with the diagnosis, prescription of inadequate doses of antidepressant medication for inadequate durations and lack of objective clinical markers.[33] The average adherence rate for long-term medication use is just over 50% in all cultures, but it is even less in those countries where health is dominated by infectious diseases that usually need only short courses of treatment. The more lengthy, complex or disruptive the medical regimen, the less likely patients are to adhere. Factors that improve adherence to treatment will include: a trusting physician–patient relationship, education of the patient regarding the goals of therapy and the consequences of good or poor adherence, a negotiated treatment plan, recruitment of family and community support, simplification of the treatment regimen and reduction of the adverse consequences of the treatment regimen.[18]

Healthcare system factors

Many of the problems associated with under-recognition and undertreatment of mental health problems are due to the healthcare system, politics, government financial constraints and lack of workforce. Addressing these issues is beyond the realm of individual health professionals but opportunities to advocate improved healthcare and human rights should not be missed.

Societal and environmental factors

Models of emotional health and well-being that take into account the local cultural, economic, familial, political, religious and social situations will be needed in different countries.[34] Stigma, cultural misunderstanding and past experiences of medical care can all affect the patient's views of medical care and if possible these should be addressed at an individual level. Funding for mental health promotion and stigma reduction is limited in most countries but again the health professional can act as an advocate in this area. Health professionals should see as part of their job the encouragement of local efforts to begin support groups, advocate to government and improve mental health literacy.

It is of the utmost importance to take into account the pathological consequences of 'racism, sexism, imperialism, colonialism, and other "isms" that produce powerlessness, marginalization, and underprivileging'.[6] Many human problems such as despair, hopelessness and helplessness are not located in the brain of the individual, but in their pattern of interaction with family, community or the wider society.[6] Individual mental health and the health of society are inextricably linked. Overwhelming social problems can not only lead to the failure of a patient to recover from their mental health problems, but can also lead to the burnout of the health professional, who may feel a strong sense of 'therapeutic impotence'. Marsella aptly says that mental health is 'not only about biology and psychology, but also about education, economics, social structure, religion, and politics'.[19] He goes on to say that the despair bred by powerlessness, the hopelessness bred by poverty, the anger and resentment bred by inequality, the low self-esteem and self-denigration bred by racism, and the confusion and conflict bred by cultural disintegration and destruction make mental health almost impossible in many places in today's world.[19]

7 CHOOSING APPROPRIATE THERAPEUTIC OPTIONS

➤ Must take into account the 'health literacy' of the patient.
➤ Must take into account the cultural expectations of both patient and health professional.
➤ Needs a strong therapeutic relationship.
➤ The health professional needs to maintain his or her own integrity whilst remaining centred on the needs of the patient.
➤ Should enable people to enhance their self-help skills, incorporating the informal family social environment as well as formal support mechanisms.[18]

The 'health literacy' of the patient and the cultural expectations of both patient and health professional are essential in the process of exploring therapeutic options (the classification and implementation of the different psychotherapies are discussed in later chapters). Mental healthcare should ultimately aim at empowerment and use efficient treatment techniques which enable people with mental disorders to enhance their self-help skills, incorporating the informal family social environment as well as formal support mechanisms.[18]

From our experience, one of the most important predictors of success in cross-cultural care is the establishment of a strong therapeutic relationship. If the patient does not understand his or her illness or management or does not trust the health professional, the treatment is unlikely to succeed. Reflective questioning, exploration of beliefs and fears, respect for differences in perception, clear explanations and proactive follow-up are all part of being interested in the person as well as the illness. If patients feel their beliefs, values and practices are understood and respected by the practitioner, there is an increased likelihood that a good relationship will be established and the patient will trust the health professional.[26] However, it is also important that the professional maintain his or her own integrity whilst remaining centred on the patient. It is a difficult balance between meeting the needs of the patient, establishing a therapeutic relationship, practising evidence-based medicine and maintaining boundaries.

All health professionals use different styles with different patients and at different stages of their illness. It is important to consider which of these styles is most appropriate according to a patient's culture as well. Styles may be authoritarian, instructional or empathic at an individual level but should also be collaborative with the family, community and management team.[35] For example, African and Afghani patients are often more used to an authoritarian or instructional style and may feel that the health professional is not confident if he or she uses only an empathic style of relating. The health professional may need to use a combination of different styles so that both health professional and patient are assured of a good outcome. So an instructional style might be appropriate if the health professional has learnt about some of the aspects of the culture, the Cultural Awareness Tool is used in an empathic manner, a community health worker is part of the team and adequate follow-up is ensured.

8 FOLLOW-UP OF THE PATIENT

➤ Review barriers if the patient does not return.
➤ Explore patient expectations of cure rather than treatment.
➤ Most people with one untreated disorder progress to develop co-morbid disorders.
➤ There are many public dimension consequences of untreated mental disorders.

Some people may be expecting a 'cure' of their illness in a short period of time. Sometimes this is because patients are more used to the acute nature of infectious diseases rather than the more chronic path of mental illness, but it is also a promise often made by charlatans.

It is important to view the barriers to access and treatment if the patient does not return. It may be something simple like lack of transport or finances. Other social determinants that are likely to influence health such as education, housing, social supports, literacy and religious beliefs may need to be reviewed. However, it may be that they don't return because of one of the other underlying patient barriers or the health professional's way of working. It may be necessary to involve the cultural mentor, traditional healer or members of the family for feedback if a patient does not return for follow-up and the health professional thinks there are cultural barriers that need to be addressed.

Some patients may continue to underestimate severity, think they can handle the episode themselves, see it as an expected response to a life situation or not see it as serious enough to continue treatment or come for follow-up.[32] Patients may view themselves as morally weak, unable to care for themselves, unable to handle responsibility, dangerous and unworthy of respect, and follow-up and long-term treatment may exacerbate these feelings.[36] It is important for the health professional to continue to support the patient, especially if stigma, shame or cultural identification with physical rather than psychological illness are barriers.

The consequences of inadequately treated mental illness are enormous and good management in any community involves more than diagnosis. Mental illness imposes a huge burden on society because of its high prevalence, underdiagnosis, undertreatment, decreased quality of life for patients and their families, high morbidity and mortality and substantial economic losses.[32] Mental disorders not only entail a higher burden than cancer, but also are responsible for more than 15% of the total burden of all diseases, nearly 15% of all DALYs (disability-adjusted life years), 12% of all disease-related mortality and 34% of all non-communicable disease DALYs.[37] Unemployment rates for people with serious and persistent psychiatric disabilities are 80–90%. As a result, people with mental disabilities constitute one of the largest groups of social security recipients. If treatment rates for the major conditions in developing countries are increased to equal those in developed countries, 26 million DALYs would be saved in 2020.[37]

Undiagnosed and undertreated mental health disorders cause antisocial and self-harming behaviours, substance misuse, 'risk-taking' behaviours, occupational impairment and problems in interpersonal and family relationships.[32] Indirect costs should also be taken into account such as premature death, absenteeism, lost productivity, pain and suffering, quality of life issues, expenses for families, hospitalisation for co-morbid physical conditions or excess tests looking for general medical diagnoses.[32] When one member has a chronic mental illness, others in the family may suffer or have to give up work and some of their social roles.[16] Patients whose depression has been correctly recognised and treated make use of healthcare services to a lesser extent and have fewer medical tests and less hospitalisation than those whose depression has not been recognised.[7,39]

Optimal mental health is not only essential for individual well-being, but also contributes to enhancing individual productivity and social cohesiveness, both of which are critical for economic growth and poverty reduction.[37] There is a high cost to employers from absenteeism and lost productivity, as mental illness often affects people in their prime working years.[32] The majority of those who are appropriately treated for depression will improve work performance and reduce disability days sufficient to offset any employer costs for treatment.[38]

The stigma attached to inadequately treated schizophrenia creates a vicious cycle of alienation and discrimination leading to social isolation, inability to work, alcohol or drug abuse, homelessness or excessive institutionalisation.[18] As well as the breaches of human rights that are often involved, imprisoning people with addiction and mental illness is almost four times more costly than treating them.[40]

A number of screening, education and treatment programmes have been shown to reduce depression in mothers and prevent adverse health outcomes such as poor cognitive development for their children.[18,41] Early intervention is fundamental in preventing progress towards a full-blown disease, in controlling symptoms and in improving outcomes. The earlier the institution of a proper course of treatment, the better the prognosis.[18] The early recognition and treatment of depression, alcohol dependence and schizophrenia are important strategies in the prevention of suicide.[18] Long periods of untreated illness may also be harmful to those with less severe disorders. Untreated mental illness has been associated with a reduction in the efficiency of immune mechanisms and with increased vulnerability to infectious disease, neoplasia and heart disease.[7]

Neural 'kindling' (Box 2.4) can cause untreated psychiatric disorders to become more frequent, severe, spontaneous and treatment refractory. Most people with one untreated disorder progress to develop co-morbid disorders, and such co-morbidity is associated with an even more persistent and severe clinical course.[15] There is a tendency by the medical profession to pay less attention to general health problems in people with mental disorders.[42] For example, depressed diabetic patients are more likely to have a poorer diet, more frequent hyperglycaemia, greater disability and higher healthcare costs than non-depressed diabetics.[18]

The public dimension consequences of untreated mental disorders include: violence, crime, homicide, juvenile delinquency, early pregnancy, excessive risk-taking, drug and alcohol abuse, self-destructive behaviour, street children, increased accidents and social neglect.[18,37]

BOX 2.4 THE PHENOMENON OF NEURAL KINDLING

If you heat with a woodstove, you know that there is a need for adequate clearance between your stove and combustibles, especially wood. Over the years, as the stove heats the wood near it, the kindling point or ignition temperature of that same wood gradually lowers because of the heat/re-heat cycle. In time, it will actually combust at a temperature much lower than before it was exposed to the heat/re-heat cycle. This is known as the kindling effect.

Similarly, if depression and anxiety are untreated or undertreated then it will take less provocation for a more severe bout of mental illness to occur in the future.[43]

9 BOUNDARIES AND SELF-CARE

➤ In many cultures there may not be a role that could be described as 'psychotherapist' or even 'general practitioner'.

➤ The health professional may be seen in the context of 'community elder' and not seen as a professional.

➤ The health professional may be vulnerable in the community if there are no firm boundaries.

➤ For those health professionals who do not have a support system of their own, finding friendship in a new community, a new culture or even a new country can be very difficult, especially in rural communities, and they may feel isolated.

➤ It is important to protect oneself from compassion fatigue and burnout.

For those health professionals who do not have a support system of their own, finding friendship in a new community, a new culture or even a new country can be very difficult, especially in rural communities. It is important that the health professional and their family have some quarantined places and time free from the medical role. This will be difficult in a small community or where there are only a few 'kindred spirits', for instance from the health professional's own culture. It is paramount to maintain the ability to laugh, exercise, sleep soundly, meditate, listen to music or practise hobbies.

For example, one of the major contributors to international medical graduates leaving rural and Aboriginal communities in Australia is their families. If the partner or children are not happy, have not found work, have inadequate education or limited social life, then the health professional is unlikely to be happy themselves.[10]

Health professionals may come from a culture or an environment where there is no system of primary care or general practice, and therefore they may be unfamiliar with these roles. Even if they have been trained as general practitioners, this may have been in a country where mental health is not integrated into primary care.

The health professional may be seen in the context of 'community elder' and not seen as a professional. This may assist in the therapeutic relationship but may make the health professional more vulnerable in the community, as there will be no firm boundaries between professional and social life. There may be a misunderstanding of the health professional's place in some cultures, with increased demands of time, paperwork, favours and gifts. If health professionals are seen as being in a rich and privileged position, patients may become angry that they are not using their money and power to assist them.

This might be a realistic expectation of a community elder in a collectivist culture but is not an appropriate role for a health professional with a patient. Liaison with other health professionals, health services, government agencies etc should be seen in the context of the professional role, with firm boundaries about confidentiality, maintenance of integrity and finances. Many patients who are not used to the role of a health professional or doctor may expect a lot more from the health professional than they are comfortable with or than is appropriate.

Protection from compassion fatigue and burnout is of the utmost importance. A chronically stressed health professional is not going to be able to deal adequately with all the cultural issues, let alone the clinical problems. Without this step, all else will come to nothing. The health professional's ability to learn will be blunted, subtle cultural issues will pass unnoticed and valuable therapeutic relationships are unlikely to blossom. To stay vigilant about self-care is difficult but essential. This means looking after physical, emotional and spiritual health.[44] A sense of humour, adequate time for relaxation, exercise, sufficient nutrition, sharing emotions with close friends, debriefing with colleagues and a balanced lifestyle generally are not added extras but are fundamental to working across cultures.

A model suggested by Karen Saakvitne and Laurie Pearlman from the Traumatic Stress Institute/Centre for Adult and Adolescent Psychotherapy in the USA addresses awareness, balance and connection in the personal, professional and organisational realms.[45] Assessing personal reactions to the confusing and sometimes overwhelming or even frightening situations may be done alone but is best done with trusted associates, with family or in a group. In some remote areas teleconferences are available for continued education, supervision and support.

Feelings such as helplessness, guilt about enjoying life, anger, irritability, overwhelming emotions, vulnerability, intolerance and disappointment with colleagues who are seen as unsupportive should be heeded. Health professionals should ensure that there are adequate safeguards for their own health and well-being and ask for help if they are at risk of suffering from burnout, compassion fatigue or vicarious trauma.[4,6]

10 EVALUATION OF THE PROCESS

➤ Part of the ongoing relationship of the health professional with the community.
➤ Evaluation may also be by the cultural mentor, community and the patients in consultation with the health professional.

➤ An evaluation of where the patient, community and health professional are in the gradual transformation of cultural dissonance through the stages of precontemplation, contemplation, planning, action and maintenance.

Everyone has their own ethnocentric outlook firmly entrenched into their personality and view of life. Motivated and perceptive health professionals can only have a glimpse into their patients' worlds as they struggle with them to help overcome their difficulties. A cultural mentor and a network from the local community will be helpful to continue to teach, support and help evaluate outcomes long-term, as the health professional can never fully understand everything about a different culture. Evaluation will help the health professional learn, and it makes the patient not only part of their own therapy, but part of the ongoing relationship of the therapist with the community. Evaluation is best done by the cultural mentor as well as by the health professional, the primary care team, individual patients and maybe by the community itself.[9]

Misunderstandings, burnout, family difficulties, financial burdens, loneliness and political pressures all mean there is often a high turnover of health professionals in cross-cultural settings. Chronic mental illness is best served by a continuity of care, and the maintenance of an experienced workforce with an established relationship with the community is vital.

Patience is a crucial virtue when working in the area of cross-cultural mental health. It may take years before patients and health professionals reach a mutual understanding about the diagnosis, treatment and prevention of mental health problems. As the patients understand more about mental health, the health professional understands more about the culture, and the therapeutic relationships will deepen. This process is likely to follow the well-known stages of change for both health professionals and patients.[47] Health professionals will progress from the precontemplative state of unconscious ethnocentrism, to the contemplative stage of seeing that different cultures might have different needs, to the planning stage of buying and reading this book, to the action of implementing the process of working across cultures and then to the maintenance of self-care and evaluation. Similarly, patients may move from having no concept of mental health, to realising that there are patterns of physical illness that may have a psychological basis, to looking for and learning about those patterns, to asking for help and finally to overcoming the barriers and continuing treatment and maintaining health. None of this is going to happen suddenly and every patient and every health professional will move through these phases at different rates and have different needs.

PRACTICAL POINTS

➤ Psychotherapy and mental health consultations across cultures will challenge a health professional's own cultural beliefs and consultation skills.
➤ Learning about cultural differences will be lifelong.
➤ More success will ensue if the health professional has patience, humility, tolerance of ambiguity, adjusts expectations and an ability to adapt behavioural style to take new culture into account.

CONCLUSION

Cultural sensitivity in consultations is ultimately about the same parameters that make for good practitioners in any situation – self-awareness, rapport, evidence-based medicine, health promotion, respect, collaboration and good communication. Keeping these values in mind will ensure that a strong therapeutic alliance will develop with more successful outcomes for both doctor and patient.[26]

It is up to the health professional to have the maturity to be adaptable, stable and able to tolerate ambiguity.[10] To maintain the humble position of a student of culture whilst adapting behaviour and psychotherapeutic techniques so as to be beneficial in different cultures is a lifelong journey. It is a delicate balance and must be evaluated regularly for negative consequences but also for the positive transformation that will ensue. The concept of 'compassion satisfaction' is a treasured outcome. It describes a sense of strength, self-knowledge, confidence, meaning, spiritual connection and respect for human resiliency. For those health professionals who work across cultures there is the potential for a unique sense of fulfilment and growth and a deeper awareness of the human condition.[48]

REFERENCES

1 Vicary D, Bishop B. Western psychotherapeutic practice: engaging Aboriginal people in culturally appropriate and respectful ways. *Aust Psychol.* 2005; **40**: 8–19.
2 Ekstrom S. The mind beyond our immediate awareness: Freudian, Jungian, and cognitive models of the unconscious. *J Anal Psychol.* 2004; **49**: 657–82.
3 Gautam M. *Irondoc: practical stress management tools for physicians.* Ottawa: Book Coach Press; 2004.
4 Dupraw M, Axner M. *Working on Common Cross-Cultural Communication Challenges.* 2001. Available at: www.pbs.org/ampu/crosscult.html (accessed January 2008).
5 Australian Bureau of Statistics. *Year Book Australia. 2008.* Available at: www.abs.gov.au/AUSSTATS/abs@.nsf/7d12b0f6763c78caca257061001cc588/F1C38FAE9E5F2B8 2CA2573D200110333?opendocument (accessed March 2008).

6 Marsella A. Culture and psychopathology. In: Kitayama S, Cohen D, editors. *Handbook of Cultural Psychology*. New York: Guilford Publications, Inc; 2007. pp. 797–818.

7 World Health Organization. *The Introduction of a Mental Health Component into Primary Health Care*. 1990. Available at: www.who.int/mental_health/media/en/40.pdf (accessed March 2008).

8 American Psychiatric Association. *Diagnostic and Statistical Manual of Mental Disorders: DSM-IV-TR*. Washington DC: APA; 1994.

9 Vicary D, Andrews H. Developing a culturally appropriate psychotherapeutic approach with indigenous Australians. *Aust Psychol.* 2000; **35**: 181–5.

10 Arkles R. *Overseas Trained Doctors in Aboriginal and Torres Strait Islander Health Services: a literature review*. 2006. Available at: www.crcah.org.au/publications/downloads/Overseas-Trained-Doctors.pdf (accessed January 2008).

11 Chhavi P, Wright B, Febbo S, *et al*. *Travelling the World Over Eight Evenings: a cross-cultural mental health training program for GPs*. 2000. Available at: www.mmha.org.au/mmha-products/synergy/Spring2000/TravellingtheWorld (accessed June 2007).

12 Vicary D, Westermann T. *'That's just the way he is': some implications of Aboriginal mental health beliefs*. Available at: www.auseinet.com/journal/vol3iss3/vicarywesterman.pdf (accessed January 2008).

13 Mckenzie A, Alberts V. *National Guidelines for the Development of Indigenous Cultural Mentors*. Townsville: James Cook University, Centre for General Practice and Rural Medicine; 2002.

14 Eckermann A, Dowd T, Chong E, *et al*. *Binan Goonj: bridging cultures in Aboriginal health*. Sydney: Elsevier Australia; 2006.

15 Vicary D, Bishop B. Western psychotherapeutic practice: engaging Aboriginal people in culturally appropriate and respectful ways. *Aust Psychol.* 2005; **40**: 8–19.

16 Wang P, Berglund P, Olfson M, *et al*. Failure and delay in initial treatment contact after first onset of mental disorders in the national comorbidity survey replication. *Arch Gen Psychiatry.* 2005; **62**: 603–13.

17 Gureje O, Alemem A. Mental health policy development in Africa. *Bull World Health Organ.* 2000; **78**: 475–82.

18 Whitley R, Kirmayer L, Groleau D. Understanding immigrants' reluctance to use mental health services: a qualitative study from Montreal. *Can J Psychiatry.* 2006; **51**: 205–9.

19 World Health Organization. *The World Health Report 2001. Mental Health: new understanding, new hope*. Available at: www.who.int/whr/2001/en/whr01_en.pdf (accessed April 2008).

20 Marsella A, Yamada A. Culture and mental health: an introduction and overview of foundations, concepts, and issues. In: Cuellar I, Paniagua F, editors. *Handbook of Multicultural Mental Health*. New York: Academic Press; 2000. pp. 3–24.

21 Benson J. *Third Culture Personalities and the Integration of Refugees into the Community: some reflections from general practice*. Available at: www.mmha.org.au/mmha-products/synergy/2003_No2/ThirdCulturePersonalities/ (accessed April 2008).

22 Kirmayer L. Culture and psychotherapy in a creolizing world. *Transcult Psychiatry.* 2006; **43**: 163–8.

23 Tamasese K, Peteru C, Waldegrave C, *et al*. Ole Taeao Afua, the new morning: a qualitative investigation into Samoan perspectives on mental health and culturally appropriate services. *Aust N Z J Psychiatry.* 2005; **39**: 300–9.

24 Group for the Advancement of Psychiatry. *Cultural Assessment in Clinical Psychiatry.* Arlington, Virginia: American Psychiatric Publishing, Inc; 2002.

25 The Transcult Psychiatry Unit, Curtin University and RACGP WA Research Unit. *Cultural Awareness Tool. Understanding Cultural Diversity in Mental Health.* Available at: www.mmha.org.au/mmha-products/books-and-resources/cultural-awareness-tool-cat/file (accessed January 2008).

26 Kleinman A, Good B, editors. *Culture and Depression: studies in the anthropology and cross-cultural psychiatry of affect and disorder.* Berkeley: University of California Press; 1995.

27 Benson J. A culturally sensitive consultation model. *Australian e-Journal for the Advancement of Mental Health.* 2006; 5(2). Available at: www.auseinet.com/journal/vol5iss2/benson.pdf (accessed April 2008).

28 Minas H, Silove D. Transcultural and refugee psychiatry. In: Bloch S, Singh B, editors. *Foundations of Clinical Psychiatry.* Melbourne, Australia: Melbourne University Press; 2001. pp. 475–90.

29 Cariceo C. Challenges in cross-cultural assessment: counselling refugee survivors of torture and trauma. *Aust Soc Work.* 1998; **51**(2): 49–53.

30 Rusch N, Angermeyer M, Corrigan P. Mental illness stigma: concepts, consequences, and initiatives to reduce stigma. *Eur Psychiatry.* 2005; **20**: 529–39.

31 Ustun T, Sartorius N, editors. *Mental Illness in General Health Care: an international study.* Chichester, England: John Wiley & Sons; 1995.

32 Tylee A, Walters P. Underrecognition of anxiety and mood disorders in primary care: why does the problem exist and what can be done? *J Clin Psychiatry.* 2007; **68**(Suppl. 2): S27–30.

33 Hirschfield R, Keller M, Panico S, *et al.* The National Depressive and Manic-Depressive Association consensus statement on the undertreatment of depression. *J Am Med Assoc.* 1997; **277**: 333–40.

34 Cohen A. *Nations for Mental Health. The Effectiveness of Mental Health Services in Primary Care: the view from the developing world.* Geneva, Switzerland: Mental Health Policy and Service Department, World Health Organization; 2002. Available at: www.who.int/mental_health/media/en/50.pdf (accessed January 2008).

35 Lloyd M. Medical authoritarianism and its effect on health care. *Med J Aust.* 1974; 2: 413–16.

36 Yen C, Chen C, Lee Y, *et al.* Self-stigma and its correlates among outpatients with depressive disorders. *Psychiatr Serv.* 2005; **56**: 599–601.

37 Gulbinat W, Manderscheid R, Baingana F, *et al.* The International Consortium on Mental Health Policy and Services: objectives, design and project implementation. *Int Rev Psychiatry.* 2004; **16**: 5–17.

38 Stuart H. Mental illness and employment discrimination. *Curr Opin Psychiatry.* 2006; 19: 522–6.

39 Lecrubier Y. Widespread underrecognition and undertreatment of anxiety and mood disorders: results from 3 European studies. *J Clin Psychiatry.* 2007; **68**(Suppl. 2): S36–41.

40 Delos Reyes C. Overcoming pessimism about treatment of addiction. *J Am Med Assoc.* 2002; **287**: 1857.

41 World Health Organization. *Mental Health Policy and Service Guidance Package. The Mental Health Context.* 2003. Available at: www.who.int/mental_health/resources/en/context.PDF (accessed April 2007).

42 Hocking B. Reducing mental illness stigma and discrimination – everybody's business. *Med J Aust.* 2003; **178**(Suppl. 9): S478.

43 New & Improved, Creating Growth through Innovation. *Energizing Curiosity in Your Innovative Brain.* 2006. Available at: www.newandimproved.com/newsletter/2035.php (accessed May 2008).

44 Snowdon T, Benson J, Proudfoot J. Capacity and the quality framework. *Aust Fam Physician.* 2007; **36**: 12–14.

45 Saakvitne K, Pearlman L. *Transforming the Pain: a workbook on vicarious traumatisation.* London: Norton; 1996.

46 Benson J, Magraith K. Compassion fatigue and burnout. *Aust Fam Physician.* 2005; **34**: 497–8.

47 DiClemente C, Prochaska J. Self change and therapy change of smoking behavior: a comparison of processes of change in cessation and maintenance. *Addict Behav.* 1982; **7**(2): 133–42.

48 Figley C, editor. *Compassion Fatigue: coping with secondary traumatic stress disorder in those who treat the traumatized.* New York: Psychology Press; 1995.

Psychotherapy across cultures

3

General principles of psychotherapy and counselling

This chapter explores:
- The nature of psychotherapy
- Common Western psychotherapeutic models
- Family therapy and group therapy
- Complementary and alternative therapies
- Traditional healers
- The clientele for psychotherapy
- Cultural views of psychotherapy
- Taboo subjects

Psychotherapy is the treatment of mental illness by psychological rather than 'medical' means such as medication.[1] The aim of any form of psychotherapy is to alleviate suffering, prolong life and reduce disability. The effectiveness of whether recovery or an improvement has taken place will vary enormously in different cultural settings.[2] Psychotherapy changes a patient's view of themselves, their relationships and their outlook by enhancing positive experiential change and neural network growth and integration.[3] This success relies on the development of a safe and trusting relationship; gaining new information and experience in thoughts, emotions, sensation and behaviour; and developing a method of processing and organising new experiences so as to continue to grow and integrate them outside therapy.[3]

Which therapies are chosen depends as much on the practitioner as on the patient. Practitioner factors are likely to include professional education, experience and cultural background. As people often consult a general practitioner (GP) as the first person in their quest for understanding and/or cure, these factors are important, as are attitudes to certain treatments and time pressures. GPs are often the gatekeepers for referral to other professionals, particularly in health services where a GP referral is needed to reduce the costs of more specialised care.

In the context of this book we need to consider to what extent it is vital that clinician and patient have a shared understanding of mental health related to their cultural backgrounds. Can cultural upbringing get in the way of the therapeutic relationship and is cultural diversity a barrier to empathy?

THE NATURE OF PSYCHOTHERAPY

The purpose of psychotherapy is to relieve psychological disability and thus ameliorate suffering by helping patients to change their attitudes and behaviour.[4] The relationship between the therapist and patient is extremely important for this process.

Communication is a key to success – the therapist must be able to help the patient explore their symptoms and problems, even if the patient is not able to verbalise these to any great extent. The patient must have belief in the potential of the therapist to effect change and feel safe to choose to discuss emotions and his or her life story, however upsetting this might be to both patient and therapist. Of course the relationship builds over time, and full disclosure may not be possible in the early stages. Without the patient trusting the doctor/therapist from the beginning, it is unlikely that the patient will return for further consultations. Language and cultural barriers may hinder the development of such trust.

While we usually give people the title psychotherapist following a structured training programme sanctioned by the health profession, a therapist may not necessarily be a professional. Indeed if thinking of the therapist as a healing agent, therapy may be provided by one or a group of fellow sufferers (self-help groups), a friend or even a book.[4]

In the age of 'evidence-based medicine', psychotherapy presents many problems in the assessment of its usefulness. As health professionals and patients become more multicultural, even more difficulties in the use of psychotherapy develop. Most 'evidence' will have been gathered using dominant-culture therapists on dominant-culture patients. The outcomes of these studies cannot necessarily be extrapolated to treatment by a dominant-culture therapist of a patient from a different culture or to treatment by an international medical graduate/health professional of a local patient. Characteristics that would usually guide a mental health diagnosis will often have very different connotations in different cultures, for example: hearing voices, seeing visions of dead relatives, attitudes to authority, sexuality, submissiveness, aggression or shame.[5]

Hopelessness, loss of meaning and loss of purpose are seen as central to the Western concept of depression. They are linked into the biopsychosocial model of disease, and treatment will often involve challenging the negative concepts using cognition or distracting from them with behavioural strategies. This may be similar to the 'loss of soul' or 'control by evil spirits or spells' that is experienced in many other cultures. If patients have no soul or have been possessed, then they too will feel hopeless and will have lost the meaning or purpose in their lives. To bring back their soul or exorcise the spirit will involve rituals and spiritual exercises that will renew meaning or purpose and change their focus to a more concrete and 'useful' way of thinking and behaving. If a patient views their problem as either spiritual or physical, cognitive and/or behavioural therapies are unlikely to be of assistance.

In many cultures the majority of the factors that influence mental health will be social and environmental. Extreme poverty, cultural collapse and disintegration, violence, homelessness, overcrowding, social isolation, rapid social change and loss of ethnic identity are all likely to lead to conflict, confusion and despair.[6]

It is always going to be difficult to choose a type of psychotherapy that will suit a particular patient but this is going to be even more of a problem when working in a cross-cultural situation. As a guide, those who have shown resilience in the past will probably benefit from a patient-focussed therapy such as narrative therapy. Those who seem to need some more skills to help them become well again may benefit from some of the cognitive behavioural therapy interventions such as sleep hygiene, breathing techniques, activity planning or problem solving. However, cognition is very much a culturally based phenomenon and assisting patients from a different culture to access negative automatic thoughts and challenge thinking errors is fraught with danger. The two parties may either consciously or unconsciously disagree on what is 'negative' or an 'error'. What is normal, morally good, acceptable, desirable, appropriate, right or true will be different in every culture.

Similarly, patients with more deep-seated psychological problems stemming from their childhood or severe trauma, who are likely to need long-term analysis of unhelpful core beliefs, will be difficult to treat across cultures. Firstly, these beliefs will usually only be accessible in their original language and so will need a highly trained interpreter. Accessing deeply held beliefs that are interfering with normal life function and challenging those beliefs as unhelpful is possible. However, the use of 'rightbrain' techniques such as hypnosis, dream analysis and art therapy may reveal cultural images that only the patient themselves will be able to interpret.

The subtleties of intonation and body language are very much culturally mediated. The interpretation of these in therapy will either need the therapist's thorough understanding of their cultural meaning or constant explanation from patient to therapist if the cultures are different. Similarly, the patient will need to learn the meaning of the therapist's body language and intonation, as these may be misinterpreted if differences are not identified. The communication of empathy, for instance, from therapist to patient will often rely on modulation of the voice, eye contact or other subtle means that may be lost across cultures.

Eclecticism in therapy

Terminology in psychotherapy can be confusing. For many practising therapists and health professionals the boundaries between the various types of therapy become blurred. Aspects are borrowed from other 'schools', and generalist practitioners, who look after the whole person's physical and psychosocial problems, are usually not trained in one particular model. Pamela Hays, an American clinical psychologist, stresses that therapists should be eclectic and flexible in their choice of therapy to reflect the cultural differences in coping strategies and management. She suggests that such eclecticism may take one of two forms: *transtheoretical,* in which diverse theories and therapies are integrated into one model; and *technical,* in which the therapist systematically chooses from an extensive menu of interventions and procedures.[7] Multicultural therapy (MCT) or transcultural therapy is 'technical eclecticism'. This is because, unlike the common psychotherapeutic models described below which start with the question 'Which therapy should be used?', Hays believes MCT begins with 'With whom is it done?'[7]

COMMON WESTERN PSYCHOTHERAPEUTIC MODELS

Western psychotherapy, as practised by qualified and registered therapists, falls into three main categories (Box 3.1). All stem from the context of mind–body separation, an idea that is alien to many other cultures.

BOX 3.1 THE THREE MAIN PSYCHOTHERAPEUTIC MODELS

- **Analytical:** Involves exploration of the patient's life and experiences, with an emphasis on the unconscious. Originally formulated by Freud; there are now many different psychoanalytical schools.

- **Patient or client-centred:** Often described as non-directive counselling; based on the work of Carl Rogers.
- **Behavioural/cognitive:** Involves exploring the effects of the immediate environment on the patient's mental processes and trying to change the patient's reactions to stimuli. Based on the work of Pavlov and Skinner. Includes behaviour modification and cognitive behavioural therapy (CBT). Sometimes called directive psychotherapy in contrast to patient-centred.

Some authorities label the analytical and patient-centred forms as 'evocative' and include these within existential therapy. Evocative therapies arise from the assumption that human beings are not getting the most out of life in terms of relationships, happiness and self-fulfilment. Existential therapy is based on philosophical doctrines, while analytical therapy concentrates on dealing with possible precipitating factors such as childhood experiences. The concept of existentialism is firmly based within the Western philosophical tradition, with its two most famous proponents being Sartre (France) and Heidegger (Germany). Therefore, existentialism would seem to have little in common with non-Western cultural beliefs, particularly as the fundamental principle is that humans become who they are because of what they do, not because of what they are born with. The existentialist view suggests that mental dysfunction arises from a patient's view that life is meaningless. Therapy is therefore aimed at helping the patient find a purpose in life.

While analytical and existential approaches take a pessimistic look at life (based on a European life philosophy), the patient-centred model is more optimistic. Arising from a North American viewpoint, patient-centred therapy aims to promote 'self-actualisation'.[2] However, all these schools are Western and individualistic in principle.

Different types of therapists tend to practise different techniques and it may be that some practitioners have skills in several or all of them. In the Western world, cognitive behavioural therapy (CBT) has collected the most evidence on its efficacy and its use is being promoted in many countries (*see* Chapter 4). However, this result may not pertain to a cross-cultural setting. Some of the advantages and disadvantages of the different therapies are discussed further below.

The following discussion of therapies includes a transcultural perspective.

Analysis

Psychoanalysis involves a long-term 'rebuilding and restructuring of the memories and emotional responses that have been embedded in the limbic system'.[8] It will be a person's first language that will house this unconscious past, their early relationships, their sense of belonging to a community, their cultural identity and their world view.[9] Accessing early memories may necessitate the use of the language of those memories. If the analysis is not in the patient's first language, emotions, dreams and memories from that time may not be able to be part of the therapy and it may not be successful in helping the patient process that part of their life. On the other hand, it may be a way for the patient to protect themselves from the trauma of those memories. If the patient gains insight into the implication of the use of different languages to access and express a variety of emotions, it may give them more control over the impact of their past or present life.

An essential alternative to struggling through a language barrier is the use of an interpreter. The translation of complex emotions by an experienced interpreter will help the patient and therapist gain deeper insight. However, there are many difficulties with the use of an interpreter in the intense environment of analysis, as there may not be direct translations of complex psychological terms or cultural phenomena and the subtle nuances of language use will usually be lost in translation.

A key component of an analytical therapeutic relationship is transference, a Western concept. First described by Sigmund Freud, transference also occurs in other types of therapy. Transference is the unconscious process by which emotions associated with a person in the patient's life, often a parent or power figure, become transferred to the therapist.[10] Such transference can be positive – the patient feels affection towards the therapist mirroring, for example, a happy childhood; or negative – hostility is felt towards the therapist. In transcultural interactions, patients who are from a minority group and are being treated by a health professional from the dominant culture may develop a transference based on the cultural divide generated by conflict between the two cultures. This is particularly likely if the patient has had previous or ongoing experience of cultural and/or racial prejudice. The therapist is thus a part of the problem as well as hopefully being able to help with a solution.[11] The therapist needs to recognise the transference and help the patient understand their feelings.

The therapist may be aware of a resistance or antagonism from the patient and interpret this as personal whereas in reality it may be culturally based. This unconscious stereotyping can of course go both ways and a therapist may develop a counter-transference based on such differences as the patient's race, age, religion, gender, sexuality, social class or culture. Therapists who are not using their own first language may equally struggle to gain a deeper understanding of issues within the therapeutic encounter because of an unconscious counter-transference that might only be able to be acknowledged in their own first language.

As each party sees the other as an individual rather than as part of a stereotyped group, and the therapeutic relationship develops, this cultural transference and counter-transference may disappear. It may, however, need to be brought into the therapy and discussed if it seems to be disrupting progression.

Patient-centred therapies

Patient, client or person-centred therapy, also known as Rogerian therapy, is an approach to counselling that places much of the responsibility for the treatment process on the patient, with the therapist having a non-directive role. Based on the work of Carl Rogers,[12] the goals of this therapy are increased self-esteem and greater openness to experience, as well as better self-understanding and lower levels of guilt and insecurity. The patient should then enjoy more positive and meaningful interpersonal relationships.

No practitioner can be expected to develop an in-depth awareness of the subtle cultural nuances of the many patients who will cross their path. If a therapist is dealing predominantly with a particular culture because they have moved to another country or they are dealing with a specific population group, they may through study, research and experience develop a deeper understanding of that culture. With these new insights they may have more success at helping patients using analytical or CBT techniques.

However, patient-centred therapies are more likely to be successful across cultures, as they do not rely on knowledge of the other culture but on a curiosity and a respect for the different beliefs of that culture. The use of the Cultural Awareness Tool (*see* Chapter 2) developed by the West Australian Transcultural Mental Health Centre can assist a therapist in identifying what is the most important issue for the patient without necessarily having a full understanding of their cultural background.[13] Then, utilising a patient-centred therapy, the patient can succeed in building a renewed sense of self that is consistent with their own hopes and beliefs.

Cognitive behavioural therapy (CBT)

As previously discussed, cognition and what is deemed to be 'normal' or appropriate behaviour are very much culturally mediated phenomena. In situations where the therapist and the patient are from different cultures, it cannot be expected that what constitutes 'negative', 'unhelpful' or 'distorted' thought patterns will necessarily be the same. Indeed, in some languages there may be no separate words for individual thinking and feeling. The patient's concept of 'self' and how they relate to their family and society will also be deeply embedded in their cultural upbringing, and the expectations of these relationships will differ between cultures. This will impact not only on the therapy itself, but also on teaching CBT to international medical graduates. It will be difficult to conceptualise the relationship between thoughts, feelings and behaviour if the patient's or the therapist's first language does not differentiate these modalities.

On the other hand, for those patients who are gradually moving away from their original cultural expectations, having a therapist who is from a different culture may help them feel more relaxed about discussing their transition. For example, women from more male-dominant societies who are choosing career or education before family may feel more confident challenging their cultural traditions if their therapist is from a different background. (For more on a modified CBT approach, *see* Chapter 4.)

FAMILY THERAPY

Family therapy is an important management strategy for people from many cultures. Families evolve implicit rules of interacting with each other that may appear to be the problems of one individual.[2] Health professionals need to be aware that the patient may have a different definition of family from their own definition. While sessions will involve members of the family together, it is also helpful to have interactions individually so that everyone involved may express his or her own views and concerns. The therapist works with the family to explore patterns of behaviour that are contributing to the problem of the patient and subsequently to try to alter the patterns to resolve the problem. There is often an issue with communication and the therapist offers a safe environment for family members to begin to communicate more effectively with each other.

Communication may be complicated by different languages spoken across generations, or younger people may find it difficult to talk freely in front of their elders. This should be acknowledged and recognised as potentially contributing to the problem. The therapist needs to be aware of the power structure within the family and work within it. To begin to understand the power relationships within a family, the ADDRESSING framework is helpful (Box 3.2).[7] In many cases a directive problem-focussed approach is needed.[7] In the case of working with couples when individuals are from different cultural backgrounds, the therapist needs to accept the values of each.

BOX 3.2 ADDRESSING POWER WITHIN FAMILIES (ADAPTED FROM HAYS[7])

- **Age:** Generational influences. In families, which generations are represented? In couples, is there a big age gap?
- **Developmental disabilities:** If a family member has such a disability, how does this affect the power balance?
- **Disabilities (acquired):** How might this have affected the power balance?
- **Religion and spirituality:** Do religious beliefs lead to one person having more power?
- **Ethnic identity:** Are there issues relating to skin colour, ethnicity or caste in multicultural families?
- **Socioeconomic status:** How is power affected by earning capacity, education, occupation?
- **Sexual orientation:** Is any member's sexual orientation an issue?

GROUP THERAPY

Group therapy brings together people who may not know each other beforehand, but share similar problems, background or experiences. It is particularly beneficial for people who have been traumatised, such as refugees and victims of domestic violence, rape and childhood sexual abuse, but it can be useful for any collection of people with a common goal or condition. The role of groups is to support, educate, provide a sense of community and connection and engender purpose and meaning in the lives of the participants. It acknowledges that there is expertise which is brought to the group setting by the participants, as well as by the therapist. It also serves to support people – each knows he or she is 'not alone', as there are others who struggle with the same issues and feelings. People may feel very isolated in their suffering and feel there is a taboo surrounding their trauma. In a group setting they can begin to dissolve the feelings of isolation, shame and stigma.[14] Many will feel safe to disclose personal stories that they may not share in a one-to-one relationship with a therapist. In a group setting individuals know they are more likely to be understood and not judged, as others who share the same experience will have been through hardship as well, whereas a therapist will not disclose this. In listening to other people's stories, new ways of dealing with difficulties will come to light.

The concept of 'mutual aid' involves group participants developing trust, intimacy and cohesion and an acceptance of others. Through shared experiences of hardship or oppression, individuals begin to see that the source of their problem is external to themselves.[15] As well as learning and listening, participants are assisting others in the group and can begin a process of emotional healing. They can cry together, learn together and laugh together.

For many patients, the concept of one-to-one counselling with a stranger is very foreign. Those from a collectivist culture, where individuals view themselves from within society, are likely to feel more comfortable working in a group situation. This is particularly important for migrants and refugees who may have limited social networks and feel culturally isolated at a time when they are very vulnerable. The relationships that develop in this environment may give participants hope that they can form other intimate relationships that are not governed by their problems. They can increase 'health literacy' and skills that are useful in a new culture and explore the gaps in their knowledge in a safe environment. An increase in self-esteem and confidence is likely to result from learning 'skills in living', and this new expertise can then be consolidated with other members of the group. Combining activities such as music, dance, art, folklore and ethnic food will also improve the healing power of the therapy.[15]

For individuals who have experienced trauma, Herman suggests there will be three stages of group therapy[14] (Box 3.3). All groups will be different and individuals within a group will progress through the stages at different rates. One of the most important aspects of group therapy is the relationship group members have with the therapist. It is he or she who establishes the environment of trust and respect and moves the group on in the complex journey through the stages.[16] A successful recovery will involve gradual progress from uncontrolled danger to personal safety, from traumatic memory to mournful remembrance and from 'stigmatised isolation to a restored connection with others'.[16] The benefits of group therapy are many, especially for those who have been traumatised. Participants are likely to have a decrease in their symptoms, increase in resilience, improvement in socialising and better adaptability to new situations.[17]

BOX 3.3 STAGES OF GROUP THERAPY[16]

1 Establish safety.
2 Focus on the story of the traumatic event – allow participants to grieve what has been lost.
3 Integration of participants back into the community with a renewed sense of purpose – trauma is externalised.

In some groups participants will be from diverse cultural backgrounds, which may be a healing process in itself or may cause tensions. Group members may be open to learning from the cultural mix and through interaction with others with different perspectives on life and different health beliefs. However, a therapist needs to be highly skilled when leading a group in which one culture predominates and where there is a minority from another background, as racism or sexism may occur.

CREATIVE AND OTHER COMPLEMENTARY AND ALTERNATIVE THERAPIES

As Western medicine has become more 'evidence-based', more patients from Western societies seem to be going to more creative and alternative healers, with some studies showing that up to 80% of Western patients with mental illness use an alternative therapy.[18] Western medicine values those characteristics of an individualistic culture (*see* Chapter 8) that tend to rely more on the 'left brain' traits such as reasoning, cognitive problem solving, logic, language and structure. The emergence of CBT and pharmacotherapy as dominant therapies reflect the importance of these to Western society. However, alternative therapies such as kinesiology, music therapy, naturopathy, psychodrama, homeopathy, art therapy, hypnosis and dream analysis are becoming more and more popular.

The right brain is the seat of such things as connection, spirituality, music, intuition, body language, art, facial expression, emotions, dreams and images. In many collectivist cultures, these are more valued than left brain features. It is the right prefrontal cortex that seems to attenuate the emotional responses that are 'fundamental to most modern psychotherapeutic methods'.[8] The right brain 'plays a superior role in the regulation of physiological, endocrinological, neuroendocrine, cardiovascular, and immune functions'.[8] It also contains the connections of the autonomic nervous system, which regulates the functions of the body's organs and mediates the somatic components of emotional states.[8] It is not unexpected then that the expression of psychopathology and the healing from traditional healers in collectivist cultures is going to be based more on right brain features.

Traumatic memories, the ability to modulate the intensity and duration of effects such as 'shame, rage, excitement, elation, disgust, panic-terror and hopeless despair' and the task of 'establishing a personally relevant universe' are all right brain functions.[8] In Western society a yearning for 'right brain healing', not being supplied by the medical profession, has led patients to abandon Western-based mental health professionals in favour of complementary and alternative practitioners. For Western practitioners to become more left and right brain balanced there needs to be a move back to the value of the therapeutic relationship, empathy, spirituality, touch and the creative therapies for Western clientele.

There is an increasing body of literature showing that the 'placebo effect', much maligned for many years, is as strong as some of the treatments used by Western practitioners for many illnesses, including depression.[19] Patients who are given placebo are different to those who are given medication or psychotherapy. They enter into a therapeutic relationship with the 'hope and expectation that their symptoms will improve' with the medication.[21] The setting, the support, the social circumstances and of course the relationship are all important in the response to placebo.[21] Changes in a patient's brain activity with placebo can also predict whether they will respond more favourably to the addition of medication.[21] In many studies these changes are noted to be in the right side of the brain.[20]

For many decades Western medicine has also tacitly acknowledged the use of 'metaphor' as a treatment modality. From Jung to Frankl, from hypnosis to art therapy, metaphor has been used to 'access a wellspring of emotions by exposing intimate connections at the deepest level of human experience'.[21] Many authors discuss their view that it is transformation at an unconscious level that brings about personality development, not conscious understanding.[22] Concepts that are difficult to put into words, such as spirituality and trauma, may only be accessible using metaphor. The safety, the direct access to the unconscious and the ability to stand separate from the material may make the use of metaphor the only therapeutic medium possible for many patients.

New forms of psychotherapy are emerging in Western health professions that attempt to balance left and right brain work. One of these is Interactive Drawing Therapy (IDT) developed by Russell Withers in New Zealand. In IDT 'the page' is used as the vehicle for building up a story or metaphor that is then layered with words. The counsellor and patient together read both the literal and metaphorical accounts, and the patient increasingly deals with material that is more and more unconscious.[22] The 'left brain focuses on factual detail, and processes data cognitively, logically and specifically, whereas the right brain takes in the big picture in a glance, and processes data affectively, experientially and situationally'.[22] The counsellor encourages the patient to retrieve layers of images, words and emotions. Transformation occurs as new insights emerge from the unconscious, new pathways are visualised and personal characteristics are discovered.

A truly holistic Western practitioner with a patient from a collectivist culture will be dealing with the left brain healing with which they are most familiar, the right brain healing with which the patient is most familiar, as well as pharmacotherapy if it is seen as appropriate. With the addition of the important 'placebo effect' and the use of herbs that may have pharmacological activity, traditional healers may also be employing a more balanced therapy of left and right brain as well as top-down (psychotherapy) and bottom-up (pharmacotherapy) treatment.

Health promotion has long used right brain techniques in community awareness programmes. Songs, pictures, cartoons, drama, puppets, games etc are used throughout the Western world to encourage health messages. In the developing world, where literacy is often low and the culture relies more on visual and creative communication, use of right brain techniques to get the message across is even more important.

BOX 3.4 CASE STUDY 1 (KEBEDESH'S STORY)

17-year-old Kebedesh came to Australia from Ethiopia with her 13-year-old brother, having been sponsored by her aunt. Her father had been killed and her mother had 'disappeared' in the war about 10 years earlier but occasional stories filtered through that the mother had been seen and that she was still alive. The children had lived in an orphanage until they came to Australia. Kebedesh spoke only Amharic but was going to school to learn English. She was sent to the health service by the school as they were concerned about her behaviour in class. She would have bouts of anger that were very difficult for the teachers to deal with.

Kebedesh's aunt confirmed that she was having outbreaks of anger at home as well – tearing up the other children's school-work, yelling at everyone, refusing to eat or locking herself in her room and not talking to anyone for days. She was also finding it difficult to know what to do.

The first consultation did not go well. Kebedesh sat looking at the wall saying in Amharic 'There's nothing wrong with me. I'm not crazy. I don't need to be here.' The interpreter was finding this behaviour difficult and was telling her she needed to be more respectful to the doctor. The doctor was alternating between asking questions, being soothing and sympathetic, and trying to leave silences hoping that Kebedesh would feel comfortable saying something else. After half an hour the doctor brought the consultation to an end and asked Kebedesh if she would like to make another appointment. Surprisingly she said yes!!

The next appointment also looked as though it was going to be frustrating, as the interpreter did not turn up and the phone service could not find any

Amharic interpreters straight away. The doctor drew a large oval on a piece of paper with a line through the middle. She drew a simple happy face on one half and the beginning of a sad face on the other. Kebedesh finished drawing the sad face with a frown and tears in the eyes. The doctor started to talk about the things that might make people happy. She started with flowers and music and drew lines to the happy face. She then drew a picture of the sun (it was 40 degrees that day) and asked Kebedesh to draw a line to where it should go. She drew a line to the sad face, looked at the doctor and they both laughed. Slowly the two parts of the face began to be filled in with a beautiful map of Ethiopia on the sad side and school and an intricate drawing of a church on the happy side. Her 7-year-old cousin was definitely on the sad side, she was very annoying and often got Kebedesh into trouble, but there was a faint line connecting her to the happy side as well. Kebedesh's mother also sat half way between with a line to the happy face and a line to the sad face. She cried as she drew the picture and the lines, acknowledging the tension and ambivalence she felt about her mother. The doctor took a photocopy of the picture as a record of the consultation and pasted it into the notes. Kebedesh took the other copy.

At the next consultation in the presence of the interpreter, the doctor asked Kebedesh what she would like to talk about. She immediately replied that she would like to discuss her mother. She spent the consultation telling the story about how her mother disappeared, about her hope that her mother would reappear one day and about how she would like to go back to Ethiopia in case her mother was still alive. She also acknowledged her anger that her mother had left her and that she had found life difficult without a mother to protect her and care for her. She said she had missed out on being a child because of the circumstances of her upbringing and this was one of the reasons for her ambivalence about her cousin. By the end of the consultation, doctor, interpreter and Kebedesh were all in tears.

She returned one more time with her aunt, who said that her behaviour was still difficult at times but was much better. Kebedesh apologised for her behaviour, which was mostly to do with minor arguments with her brother and cousin. She said she was happy, would work hard at school, and that she was going to immerse herself more in Ethiopian music and in her church. She knew that these were the things that would make her happy if the homesickness for Ethiopia and the grief for her mother became unbearable. She said that she knew that she would always carry her mother's memory with her and that she would try to behave in a way that would make her proud of her. She promised to return if she needed to talk to the doctor again.

TRADITIONAL HEALERS

Many Western-trained health professionals are now becoming more open to the idea of working with, or at least knowing about, traditional healers. The term is more respectful than many in usage, such as medicine man, witch doctor or sorcerer (as well as quack). Shaman is another word that has a tinge of mystery about it – but could be seen as racist if only applied to healers practising in cultures viewed as primitive by some.[22] The original shamans came into being in Siberia but the word is now used for healers from other traditions.

Medical systems can be classified as internalising or externalising. Internalising systems locate the origin as well as the solutions of the problem inside the individual's body, mind or spirit. It may be toxins, germs, memories or evil spirits that need to be neutralised, destroyed or removed. It may be something such as vitamins or vital energy that is missing or depleted and must be added. It may be energy or 'wind' that is blocked and needs to be allowed to flow. Or it may be a lack of balance, as in yin/yang, that needs to be brought back into balance. Externalising medical systems locate the cause as well as the solution outside the person in the interpersonal, social or spiritual realm. Resolution will involve rituals that involve the family or community, and healing will be felt by the whole group.[2] Many indigenous people of countries such as Australia and Canada are likely to have mental health problems associated with the history of colonisation of the country and from the rapid cultural change that has ensued. Healing rituals and traditional ceremonies are likely to be a powerful force as people assert their indigenous identity in the face of assimilation and cultural disintegration and take them back to the respect for land and environment that is an essential part of the communal healing.[2]

The traditional healers and elders of many cultures have often been performing 'psychotherapy' for many generations. If there is unusual behaviour, an insoluble problem, anxiety, nightmares, depression or somatic symptoms, patients will often go to a traditional healer before they come to a health professional. This is even more likely to occur for these problems than it would for physical illness. On some occasions the patient will receive advice and on other occasions a ritual may be performed. The psychological problem may be expressed as a spiritual issue and so require a spiritual solution. Some traditional healers may even suggest medication such as herbal remedies, anti-epileptics or antidepressants. In Western countries patients will often visit alternative health practitioners or take over-the-counter medication before they see a health professional.

It is impossible to tease out the effects of symbols, rituals, psychological attitudes, expectations and any physical interventions that may take place. The effect on physiology, psychology, emotions and hence pain and healing is important in any form of therapy and will be mediated in both the left and right side of the brain.[2] For instance, a Chinese patient is likely to visit a traditional herbalist or feng shui master, who may listen to the symptoms, work out possible solutions, advise 'hot' or 'cold' food, perform acupuncture, give herbs, advise changing the environment and/or advise attending to their ancestors' graves.[24]

There is a body of research that shows that respectful 'active listening' is as beneficial as formal psychotherapy for those with mild to moderate anxiety and depression. In a country where primary healthcare professionals, psychologists and psychiatrists are in short supply, 'active listening' by an experienced and well-respected traditional healer or elder is more likely to be of benefit to the patient than a rushed consult with a time-poor health professional from a different culture. Storytelling by the healer with the 'patient' as listener may also be helpful. The story is often metaphorical with a message that may help the healing process.

Acknowledging and respecting the part that traditional healers, elders and alternative health practitioners play in the mental health of the community is difficult for many health professionals. Some skills may be able to be learnt and adapted by doctors and nurses, but others may not and the two traditions need to be able to work together for the benefit of the patient. A difficulty, of course, is that a traditional healer will not always be accessible in the migrant's new country.

BOX 3.5 CASE STUDY 2 (MAGGIE'S STORY – BACK PAIN OR DEPRESSION?)

Maggie was one of the 'Stolen Generation' – children of Australian Aboriginal descent who were taken from their mothers and put into foster homes or institutions. She had grown up without knowing who her real mother was or where her 'country' was. As an adult she found these things out but had never visited the people in the desert where she was born.

She came to the doctor because she had hurt her back at work. After six months it was still causing her many problems. She wasn't sleeping well, was hardly going out at all, was irritable most of the time, wasn't eating well and felt that her back pain was running her life. The doctor sent her to a psychiatrist, who diagnosed her with depression and suggested she take antidepressants.

Maggie didn't believe she had depression but that it was her back that was causing all her symptoms. She was still being paid by the Workcover insurance and under pressure to return to work.

Maggie became frustrated with the whole system and went to visit some relatives in the country. A ngankari (traditional Aboriginal healer) was staying nearby and Maggie went to see him. He did not speak any English and Maggie didn't speak his traditional language. However, he sang to her, lightly massaged her back and drew pictures in the dirt. Maggie felt no pain in her back during the month she was staying in the country and said she was 'back to her old self'.

On coming back to the city she tried to go back to work but her previous symptoms returned almost immediately. Her doctor called a case conference with the psychiatrist, the insurance company, the workplace, Maggie and her support people. After much discussion everyone agreed that Western medicine was not doing Maggie any good at all and that perhaps the only hope of her recovering was to spend some time in the far north of the country under the care of a ngankari.

A year later the doctor saw Maggie again. She was happy and well and was making a living selling traditional-style paintings in a town close to the city.

IS THE CHOICE OF PSYCHOTHERAPEUTIC APPROACH IMPORTANT?

The benefits of psychotherapy may not be related to the specific approach of a particular school but rather to the common factors involved in therapy, such as the therapeutic alliance, active listening by the therapist, the trust between patient and practitioner and the adherence of the patient to an agreed management plan.[25] The confidence of the patient in the therapist's explanation of the problem is of utmost importance. This explanation must take into account the patient's belief system or world view. As is the case with physical illness, without such trust the patient is unlikely to adhere to any treatment prescribed. Thus it is also important there that is a connection in the patient's mind between the explanation and the treatment. Making this connection and exploring management options are central to shared decision-making and henceforth adherence within a consultation. 'Approaching therapy through a contextual model embraces a multicultural counselling perspective.'[25] (p. 223). Such an approach is appropriate and relevant to all patient/professional interactions, as culture is not the only distinguishing attribute amongst patients seeking help (Box 3.6).

BOX 3.6 CONTEXTUAL PSYCHOTHERAPY

'. . . ideally therapists should select for each patient the therapy that accords, or can be brought to accord, with the patient's personal characteristics and view of the problem . . . therapists should seek to learn as many approaches as they find congenial and convincing. Creating a good therapeutic match may involve both educating the patient about the therapist's conceptual scheme and, if necessary, modifying the scheme to take into account the concepts the patient brings to therapy.'[2] (p. 15)

(Of course explanations, connection and shared decision-making are more problematical for patients and therapists when there is a diagnosis of severe mental illness or psychosis, but these situations are not part of the focus of this book.)

BOX 3.7 CASE STUDY 3 (THE BRAZILIAN DOCTOR – RENDER UNTO CAESAR THE THINGS THAT ARE CAESAR'S . . .)
(WITH THE KIND PERMISSION OF DR SANDRA FORTES)

It was late at night when the nurses called saying that one of the patients in the female ward was agitated and was not letting the others go to sleep. The overworked psychiatry resident found all the other patients gathered around as the woman writhed on the ground in extreme distress. She had fallen to the ground and a deep voice came from her mouth saying that 'this horse has to suffer'. The doctor, wanting to go to sleep, got near the patient and asked for the 'voice' to identify itself. The voice gave the name of one of the entities from the Brazilian African–Catholic religion: Umbanda. The voice said that the patient was not fulfilling her obligations towards her deities and because of that she had to suffer, and that was the reason she was brought to the hospital. Finally, the doctor had enough. She kneeled and told the spirit that this was her ward and that there was no place for him here. She said that doctors don't go prescribing in religious centres, so spirits should not come to hospitals, and demanded that the spirit leave the hospital immediately. To the doctor's relief and amazement the woman settled and suddenly woke up and asked what was going on. She was medicated for the night with benzodiazepine so that everybody could go to sleep. In the following days she was subsequently able to engage in supportive psychotherapy, when her personal problems, including those with her religion, were discussed. She recovered during her short stay in the hospital and when she left she went back to the Umbanda Centre and had no further problems with spirits.

THE CLIENTELE FOR PSYCHOTHERAPY

Many people brought up in developed countries, certainly within the last half century, will understand the concept of psychotherapy to some extent. This may be secondary to the pervasive influence of United States culture permeating to other countries through film and television programmes. For example, though the USA has only 4% of the world's population, its psychologists dominate the field such that non-American influenced concepts and therapies are labelled 'indigenous psychologies'.[26] In particular the notion that 'film stars' and celebrities are undergoing psychoanalysis, often for many years (for example Woody Allen), has helped to some extent to demystify the procedure. The popularised and 'dumbed down' reduction of Freudian psychotherapy as a means to sort out one's psychosexual problems is commonly alluded to in the media. However, the amusement arising from a Freudian slip is not encountered as often as was the case in the 1960s and 1970s. One of the popular ideas of psychotherapy is perhaps the patient lying on a couch pouring out the ups and downs of their life, while the therapist interjects a few words to facilitate the flow.

This Americanisation of psychoanalysis may perhaps lead to an idea that such therapy is only for the rich and famous. However, patients are familiar with the less exotic treatment of counselling and in certain circumstances are amenable to being referred for such management. Counselling was probably first seen as related to 'marriage counselling'. Now it is accepted as a management option for a wide range of problems, including alcohol and drug abuse, post-traumatic stress and relationship difficulties. TV audiences are familiar with reports, following a traumatic death or accident, of affected school children, families and professionals being offered counselling to help them cope with their thoughts and feelings.

Such readily available and, in many cases, free or subsidised counselling is unusual in other cultures. Patients from developing countries who have had trouble paying for or even accessing medical care may find the concept of 'talking cures' alien. Therefore, both foreign patients and doctors may not be aware of the services on offer or their efficacy in providing support and treatment. Considering the nature of mental health problems, the idea that treatment is necessary for patients with psychosis is likely to be accepted by most people, with the proviso that 'psychosis' needs to be defined within context. Psychosis is likely to be treated by psychiatrists and not, at least at first, within the community. Patients presenting with what used to be called neurosis – mild to moderate depression, psychosomatic illnesses and anxiety – are likely to be treated with medication. This is more likely to occur if an attempt at psychotherapy seems impossible because of communication difficulties. Some of these patients may also be over-investigated in the search for a physical cause for their symptoms. People who have left their own country and are having difficulty coping because of life events such as bereavement and relationship problems may not realise that there is help. On the other hand, they may not be managed optimally if the doctor does not recognise that such problems are legitimate as presenting problems to a clinician. Patients with alcohol and/or drug addictions may be considered empathically or as self-abusers depending on their background and the background of the health professional with whom they consult.

Refugees and migrants into developed countries may have physical and psychological problems very different to those of the patients that their doctors usually treat. Likewise, doctors trained within different cultures and themselves the victims of hardship and discrimination may have difficulty accepting that certain mental health problems of patients who appear to have no major life traumas are worthy of medical consideration.

CULTURAL VIEWS OF PSYCHOTHERAPY

Mental illness generates a certain amount of fear in most cultures. The mind has a mystery and power about it, whatever part of the body is perceived as housing the 'spirit' of the person's life, be it the kidneys, the liver, the heart or the brain. Each culture will have established boundaries of 'normal' thought processes and behaviour. They will also have ascribed meanings and causes for those who think and behave outside such boundaries. Those who in one culture may be labelled as mentally ill, in another culture may be viewed as witches, holy men, sages, prophets or just plain eccentric. For those outside the culture to describe such people as unwell and needing 'treatment' is obviously inappropriate.

Psychiatry is a new discipline in many countries and those who choose it as a career may also be ostracised by their peers. In Nepal, for example, the psychiatrists also deal with neurological conditions such as epilepsy, and the approach to psychiatric illness is similarly physical. Medication is the mainstay of treatment and, in a country of 25 million people and only 40 psychiatrists, patients need to have very severe illness to be seen. In many countries there is no middle ground between a bio-physical model of mental illness needing medication and a supernatural understanding needing spiritual intervention. Psychotherapy may be virtually untaught in any health profession, as it seems there is no place for it in the way the society conceptualises mental illness. This means that health professionals who are trained in these countries will not only have minimal understanding or training in psychotherapy, but are also likely to carry the society's deeper cultural beliefs about mental illness unconsciously. Learning psychotherapeutic techniques will involve 'unlearning', or at least being aware of, the cultural values that have informed their understanding of mental illness and its treatment. Similarly, health professionals hoping to use evidence-based psychotherapeutic techniques in patients with mental illness may strike many barriers if patients are expecting only medication, see their 'illness' as physical or spiritual, or are unfamiliar with the psychological concepts used in the therapy.

TABOO SUBJECTS

Western-trained health professionals are accustomed to patients discussing 'anything'. It is certainly expected that for counselling or psychotherapy to be successful the patient will disclose the issues that are concerning them and that they will answer the practitioner's questions. Therapies such as psychoanalysis hope to assist the patient in uncovering the deeper meanings of their thoughts, feelings or behaviour and this will usually involve discussions about past trauma, difficulties and other events. CBT involves looking at the current circumstances and unravelling the feelings, thoughts and behaviours associated with what is occurring. Even simple psychotherapies such as 'active listening' involve empathy and understanding as the basis for the therapeutic alliance and for the patient's improvement.

For many women the shame of rape, child abuse or domestic violence means that they may never speak about what happened to them, especially to a male. Many people who have been tortured, exposed to severe trauma or have post-traumatic stress disorder (PTSD) may be unable to find the words to express how they feel or what happened to them, especially in a second language. The horror of what happened remains only as images and sensations which no words could possibly convey. They are even less likely to talk about such things if there is a cultural gap causing them to fear being misunderstood or judged because of their experiences.

Indigenous cultures may have strict taboos about 'rites of passage' ceremonies. The secrecy surrounding these events can cause enormous anxiety in some people and the trauma that might occur can lead to PTSD. However, the details of what happens and sometimes even the fact that it has happened are unlikely to be discussed with the practitioner. It is very important that this is respected and the patient treated without being expected to reveal information that is culturally prohibited. The anxieties surrounding pregnancy and the trauma of labour may have similar 'women's business' taboos, only to be discussed with older women.

Many cultures have either explicit or implicit taboos about relationships and about confidentiality. Sometimes a good therapeutic relationship might involve the breaking down of these taboos and the loss of the health professional's gender, religion, age, class or dress code. This is likely to take time and patience and may be an unconscious process.

CULTURALLY APPROPRIATE PSYCHOTHERAPEUTIC PRACTICE

In Australia there have been calls for specialist mental health services for indigenous men, women and children.[27] Such advocacy arises from the complex cultural, historical and social issues of indigenous people. Culturally appropriate counselling is important but not always available for each and every minority group. Where such services are lacking, indigenous people, for example, will try other sources of help and will access 'Western' practitioners only when there are no such other options available.[28] This is likely to happen with other patient groups as well. Australian psychologists David Vicary and Brian Bishop, who undertook a qualitative study of Aboriginal health beliefs in relation to mental health, suggest that the reason for this behaviour arises from such health beliefs. Aboriginal people have a concept of wellness which can be defined as holistic, incorporating physical, mental, cultural and spiritual components.

PRACTICAL POINTS

➤ Trust is a central part of the patient–therapist relationship – language and cultural barriers may hinder the development of such trust.
➤ Western psychotherapy tends to work within the context of mind-body separation.
➤ Patient-centred therapies are more likely to be successful across cultures, as they do not rely on knowledge of the other culture but on a curiosity and a respect for the different beliefs of that culture.
➤ Western-trained health professionals need to become more open to the idea of working with, or at least knowing about, complementary therapies and traditional healers.
➤ Respectful 'active listening' is as beneficial as formal psychotherapy for those with mild to moderate anxiety and depression.
➤ Many cultures have either explicit or implicit taboos about discussing relationships and about confidentiality.

REFERENCES

1 Soanes C, Stevenson A, editors. *Oxford Dictionary of English*. 2nd ed. Oxford: Oxford University Press; 2003.

2 Kirmayer L. The cultural diversity of healing: meaning, metaphor and mechanism. *Br Med Bull*. 2004; **69**: 33–48.

3 Ekstrom S. The mind beyond our immediate awareness: Freudian, Jungian, and cognitive models of the unconscious. *J Anal Psychol*. 2004; **49**: 657–82.

4 Frank JD, Frank JB. *Persuasion & Healing: a comparative study of psychotherapy*. Baltimore: John Hopkins University Press; 1993.

5 Group for the Advancement of Psychiatry. *Cultural Assessment in Clinical Psychiatry*. Arlington, Virginia: American Psychiatric Publishing, Inc; 2002.

6 Marsella A. Culture and psychopathology. In: Kitayama S, Cohen D, editors. *Handbook of Cultural Psychology*. New York: Guilford Publications, Inc; 2007. pp. 797–818.

7 Hays PA. *Addressing Cultural Complexities in Practice*. 2nd ed. Washington: American Psychological Association; 2008.

8 Shore A. Advances in neuropsychoanalysis, attachment theory, and trauma research; implications for self psychology. *Psychoanal Inq*. 2002; **22**: 433–84.

9 Tamasese K, Peteru C, Waldegrave C, *et al*. Ole Taeao Afua, the new morning: a qualitative investigation into Samoan perspectives on mental health and culturally appropriate services. *Aust N Z J Psychiatry*. 2005; **39**: 300–9.

10 Freud S. *Outline of Psychoanalysis* (1938) with *New Introductory Lectures on Psychoanalysis* (1933). Translated by Helena Ragg-Kirkby. London: Penguin Modern Classics; 2003.

11 D'Ardenne P, Mahtani A. *Transcultural Counselling in Action*. 2nd ed. London: Sage; 1999.

12 Rogers C. *Client-Centered Therapy*. Boston: Houghton Mifflin; 1951.

13 Seah E, Tilbury F, Jayasuriya P, *et al*. *The Cultural Awareness Tool: understanding cultural diversity in mental health*. Perth: Transcultural Mental Health Network; 2001. Available at: www.mmha.org.au/mmha-products/books-and-resources/cultural-awareness-tool-cat/file (accessed March 2008).

14 Herman J. *Trauma and Recovery*. New York: Basic Books; 1992.

15 Williams J, Nesci P. *Building Resilience and Shared Journeys – A Group Therapy Model for Working with Newly Arrived Refugee Women*. Adelaide: Women's Health Statewide and The Migrant Health Service; 2005.

16 Cariceo C. Challenges in cross-cultural assessment: counselling refugee survivors of torture and trauma. *Aust Soc Work*. 1998; **51**: 49–53.

17 Nicholson B, Kay D. Group treatment of traumatized Cambodian women: a culture-specific approach. *Soc Work*. 1999; **44**: 470–9.

18 Wang P, Lane M, Olfson M, *et al*. Twelve-month use of mental health services in the United States. *Arch Gen Psychiatry*. 2005; **62**: 629–40.

19 Mayberg H, Silva J, Brannan S, *et al*. The functional neuroanatomy of the placebo effect. *Am J Psychiatry*. 2002; **159**: 728–37.

20 Arehart-Treichel J. Placebo-based brain changes affect depression outcome. *Psychiatr News*. 2006; **41**(17): 30.

21 Stone C, Everts H. The therapeutic use of metaphor in interactive drawing therapy. *N Z J Couns*. 2006; **26**(4): 31–43.

22 Withers R. Interactive drawing therapy: working with therapeutic imagery. *N Z J Couns.* 2006; **26**(4): 1–14.

23 Fernando S. Mental Health, Race and Culture. 2nd ed. Basingstoke: Palgrave; 2002.

24 Chan B, Parker C. Some recommendations to assess depression in Chinese people in Australasia. *Aust N Z J Psychiatry.* 2003; **38**: 141–7.

25 Wampold BE. *The Great Psychotherapy Debate: models, methods and findings.* New Jersey: Lawrence Erlbaum Associates; 2001.

26 MacLachlan M. Culture, empowerment and health. In: Murray M, editor. *Critical Health Psychology.* Basingstoke: Palgrave Macmillan; 2004. pp. 101–17.

27 Swan P, Raphael B. *Ways Forward: national consultancy report on Aboriginal and Torres Strait Islander mental health.* Canberra: Office of Aboriginal and Torres Strait Islander Health; 1995.

28 Vicary DA, Bishop BJ. Western psychotherapeutic practice: engaging Aboriginal people in culturally appropriate and respectful ways. *Aust Psych.* 2005; **40**: 8–19.

4

Modified cognitive behavioural therapy (CBT)

This chapter explores:
- ■ The nature of CBT
- ■ CBT and cultural concerns
- ■ Dealing with physical symptoms of mental distress
- ■ Motivational interviewing and other techniques to change thinking
- ■ Somatisation

Cognitive behavioural therapy (CBT) is used extensively in Western medicine to treat mild to moderate depression, anxiety disorders and other mild to moderate mental illness. CBT is an evidence-based and structured form of therapy that patients can also use in a self-help way. It aims to change unhelpful thinking (i.e. cognition) and behaviour.

THE NATURE OF AND RATIONALE FOR CBT

'Cognitive distortions', that is, automatic thinking errors, affect how a patient sees themselves, their world and their future. People with depression tend to have a negative view of themselves with low self-esteem, feel their world is making impossible demands on them and see their future as hopeless. Those with anxiety tend to see themselves as vulnerable, the world as high risk and their future as unpredictable. CBT is based on the idea that this distorted, negative and maladaptive thinking causes mood disturbance. The health professional's task is to help the patient access the negative thoughts that have led to the unrealistic and unhelpful emotions and to challenge those thoughts with a more realistic and helpful view of what's happening.

What constitutes 'negative' or 'threatening' will depend on the patient's upbringing, past experience and, of course, culture in the broader sense of the term. Similarly, what constitutes 'psychological dysfunction' will differ in different cultures. For the health professional who is from a different culture, negotiating the difficulties of diagnosing and then communicating the diagnosis of a mental health problem is problematic. To try to help the patient to access unconscious reasons why the emotional problem has occurred and then to challenge those, without taking an ethnocentric stance, is extremely difficult. It is probably only really possible if health professionals are constantly evaluating their own cultural views on the issues in question and have a very good understanding of their patients' cultural practices and beliefs.

Thus CBT draws on the concepts of perception, cognition, emotion and behaviour to explore how individuals perceive and respond to external and internal stimuli, how they think about that stimuli, how they react emotionally and how all this determines their behaviour. CBT relies on the individual as separate from their social situation and relies on the power of the mind being of more importance than the body, relationships, society or spirit.[1]

CBT IN TRANSCULTURAL CONSULTATIONS

CBT has become the psychotherapy with the most 'evidence' of therapeutic effectiveness and hence is the psychotherapy that is the most funded and taught across the Western world. Most of the research that has been carried out focuses on situations where both the health professional and patient are from the same culture and, like most such research, within a Western framework in the Western world. The relevance of CBT in cross-cultural consultations and in the developing world is controversial, as an emphasis on the importance of private thought processes and personal responsibility belongs to an individualistic world view. For Australian Aboriginal people, 'social and emotional well-being' is the preferred term, as even 'mental health' implies an individualistic view and does not acknowledge the social and cultural aspects. Languages of collectivist cultures may not have separate words for individual thoughts and emotions, but emotions may be expressed more in terms of relationship to family, group or community. In some Australian Aboriginal languages there is not even a word that directly translates to 'health'. Well-being is described in terms of 'happiness, land, law, strength and social responsibility'.[2]

Health professionals who have experience with CBT and have a good relationship with their patient may be able to discuss the cross-cultural differences that are likely to interfere with the therapy and acknowledge the patient as the expert in their culture. An exploration of negative automatic thoughts might then be possible using questions such as 'What real evidence is there that what you are saying is true?', 'What are the other alternatives?' or 'Is thinking this way helpful?' The discussion becomes much more patient-centred and the therapist would need to take the attitude of an inquisitive bystander with questions about the problem such as 'Who (is around), what (else is happening), when (does the problem happen), where (are you when it happens), how (does it happen) . . .?' Both patient and health professional can build up a picture together of the true nature of the problem by delving into its meaning from the patient's perspective. Some patients may find this style of questioning quite aggressive and intrusive. The health professional will need to be aware that this may be the case and be alert for reticence on the part of the patient.

The answers about what is actually realistic or helpful in the patient's culture may need input from someone else such as a community health worker, cultural mentor or patient advocate if neither patient nor health professional is able to find the solution. This consultation would need to be done with the patient's permission or the patient themselves may need to ask someone from their own culture for assistance. If the health professional is working in a community where there is a good relationship with a traditional healer, this may be an opportunity for the two professionals to work together for the added benefit of the patient.

CBT also lends itself to the exploration of cultural problems the patient may be having if they are now living in another culture. Some practices that are acceptable in one culture may be unacceptable or offensive in another and the reactions of new friends and onlookers may surprise, confuse or even depress the patient. For instance, in China spitting on the ground is very common and is not seen as offensive, in desert cultures people are not used to washing every day, Western women are used to shaking hands with men as a greeting or Middle Eastern men might hug and kiss each other when they meet. Challenging the patient's thoughts that they are being rejected and not seen as worthwhile by the new community can lead to a discussion about the problem stemming from different practices in the new culture rather than something personal about the patient. The patient is then able to decide if they are going to change their behaviour to suit the new culture or if they are going to continue their behaviour and try not to take personally any comments or 'looks' they receive.

PSYCHOLOGICAL DISTRESS AND PHYSIOLOGICAL RESPONSE

The triggers for psychological distress are likely to be different across cultures. However, the physiological responses such as the 'fight or flight' response to adrenaline, hyperventilation, insomnia, lack of motivation and fatigue will be similar. Behavioural strategies rely on challenging and working with the physiological symptoms and signs rather than their causes. On the other hand, emotions, cognition and the use of language are very culturally mediated and there is a risk that the health professional's view of what is normal, good, useful or right will differ from that of the patient.

There are many other useful strategies that come under the banner of CBT. These will include techniques that assist the patient in settling the physical symptoms of depression and anxiety (Box 4.1).

BOX 4.1 TECHNIQUES FOR DEALING WITH PHYSICAL SYMPTOMS

- Stress reduction.
- Slow breathing exercises.
- Relaxation techniques.
- Sleep hygiene.
- Activity planning.
- Mindfulness (multisensorial awareness of the present moment).

The reader is referred to a book on CBT if they are not familiar with these – see end of the chapter for suggested reading. If both health professional and patient are in agreement that the symptoms are unpleasant and unhelpful, then training in these techniques will be of assistance as part of the patient's management plan. For instance, an author from Sierra Leone suggests that harming agents such as witchcraft or curses may sometimes be able to be kept at bay with rituals that might include breathing and relaxation training.[3] In Malaysia, CBT has been modified for use within a religious framework using the Qu'ran and Hadith as guidelines and in Sri Lanka it has been modified for use with medically unexplained complaints.[4]

BOX 4.2 CASE STUDY 1 (EMERGENCY ROOM IN NEPAL)

It was a busy day in the Emergency room in the hospital in Nepal. The Australian doctor walked in to see if she was needed in any way. One of the registrars waved at a patient who did not seem to be dying but was very distressed and asked if the doctor would see if she could do anything with the patient. A very frustrated medical student was yelling at a female patient in her mid-30s, who was hyperventilating and had developed spasms in her hands and her throat. They were both obviously extremely upset and the situation was escalating rapidly. With no language in common the doctor took the patient's hand, put her other hand on her chest and quietly said 'Breathe in, breathe out' in a slow, rhythmic fashion, mimicking this as she went. Gradually the patient matched her breathing pace with the doctor's, her spasms settled and the look of fear went from her eyes. She smiled at the doctor, obviously pleased that she had been able to control the situation. The student was surprised that this had happened so quickly and without a word of Nepali being spoken. The doctor gave the medical student a quick tutorial on slow breathing exercises and how they can empower the patient to have control over panic attacks. The medical student then returned to the Emergency Department and taught the patient's relative how to help the patient slow down her breathing next time she was having a panic attack.

This patient presented in a very similar manner to a woman with tetanus who had come in the previous week with similar spasms. In a country where tetanus is still common, the tetany induced by hyperventilation is even more frightening.

CHANGING THINKING – ALTERING COGNITION

CBT has also taken on board ways of helping patients change how they think more gradually and without using the blunt line of questioning that is used when challenging negative thinking (Box 4.3).

BOX 4.3 TECHNIQUES TO HELP CHANGE THINKING

- Psychoeducation.
- Motivational interviewing.
- Structured problem solving.

Psychoeducation involves explaining to patients the connection between how they feel and their physical symptoms and signs. This is particularly useful for patients who have limited health literacy or who present with only physical symptoms rather than describing their emotions or mood. Linking the current neuropsychiatric understanding of mental illness with how a person thinks and feels may expand on this at a future consultation. Similarly, a discussion about how medication affects the brain's neurotransmitters may be helpful in encouraging a patient to continue their medication. The psychological and physical benefits of psychotherapeutic techniques and how they are measurable with psychometric tools and with brain scanning may also be part of these discussions if the health professional thinks this would be useful in the patient's understanding of their mental health issues.

Motivational interviewing acknowledges that patients do not tend to thank a health professional straight away for their insights and then immediately change their behaviour. This technique was introduced in the 1980s and refined by Miller and Rollnick in 1991.[5] It is based on the five stages of change model (Box 4.4).[6]

BOX 4.4 FIVE STAGES OF CHANGE MODEL

1 **Precontemplation:** The patient has no intention of changing their behaviour in the foreseeable future. The patient is perhaps unaware that there is a problem.
2 **Contemplation:** The patient is aware that a problem exists and is thinking about changing their behaviour but has no firm commitment to take action.
3 **Preparation:** The patient intends to change and develops a plan and a time-frame for its implementation.
4 **Action:** The patient begins to modify their behaviour to overcome the problem. This requires considerable commitment and energy.
5 **Maintenance and relapse prevention:** The patient works to prevent relapse. This stage may last for many months or years.

These five stages are probably reflective of the neurological changes that are happening as the neurons that established old thoughts and habits are changed to new pathways in the brain and gradually become stronger. It is particularly useful for people whose behaviour is detrimental to their health, such as those who smoke or drink to excess. Patients will be in the precontemplation phase if they have no cultural or personal concept of mental illness or have never realised that their unconscious thoughts can influence their mood, relationships or physical health. It is only after they have 'contemplated' what they have been told that they can start to plan what changes are possible and make decisions about what they will do, such as whether to take medication or undertake therapy with a psychologist. The health professional needs to be aware of what stage the patient is at and support and educate them appropriately. If there are barriers to moving through the stages, the health professional will need to discuss these. For patients who are from collectivist cultures, for instance, decisions might usually be made with the involvement of other important people or after consultation with a traditional therapist or religious elder.

Structured problem solving is another technique that can assist the patient in having more control over what is happening in their life without the health professional necessarily fully understanding the cultural issues at stake.[7] It involves several steps (Box 4.5).

BOX 4.5 STEPS IN PROBLEM SOLVING

- Define the problem.
- Make a list of all possible solutions.
- Evaluate the solutions according their advantages and disadvantages.
- Choose the best possible solution.
- Plan how to carry it out by breaking it down into steps.
- Review the progress.

The problem is defined by the patient, not the health professional, and similarly the solutions are only those that the patient comes up with, possibly with the help of family and community. The health professional is only acting as a guide in the process and supports and encourages the patient. The problem, the solutions, the advantages and disadvantages and how the patient carries out the plan may be completely foreign to the health professional. The review can move the process into another problem-solving exercise if the outcome has not been successful in the patient's eyes. The biggest difficulty for the health professional is to support the patient to find their own solution without the health professional's active input. Again an acknowledgement at the beginning of the difference in cultures and how this is likely to impact the process is important.

BOX 4.6 CASE STUDY 2 (PETER'S STORY)

Peter, a local Aboriginal man, had just been let out of jail, where he had been for the last three years for assaulting someone when he was drunk. He had come to the doctor for a repeat of olanzepine, a medication used for schizophrenia.

He'd taken this for the last six months while he was in jail, as he had become very distressed, not sleeping at night, and had told the prison doctor about all the dead people who were talking to him. The medication had helped him sleep and he was feeling calmer but he said it hadn't stopped the people talking. He often drank too much in order to try to block out these voices but this just made them worse when he was sober. The doctor asked him to tell her about the people and what they were saying.

Peter said that this wasn't something he was used to talking about but that he would think about it and come back later. He returned two months later with a minor illness and the doctor again asked him if he would like to talk about the voices of the dead people. She asked him if he'd ever seen anyone die.

Peter then told a long story about the 10 people he'd seen die, beginning with his grandfather being shot in front of him when he was three and ending with another Aboriginal man being purposefully crushed to death by a washing machine while he was in prison. His mother had hung herself while in custody when he was eight and he had held his beloved grandmother's hand as she died six years ago of kidney failure at the age of 48. He had never known his father.

Peter said he felt guilty that he couldn't save any of them, that he missed them and that it felt like they were all angry with him for not avenging their deaths. The doctor asked if they were telling him these things when they talked to him. He said they weren't saying these things – this was just how he felt. He said that mostly they were just saying that even though they were dead they were still there with him.

Peter had never before discussed the overwhelming grief he felt for these important people. He was also upset that he had missed some of their funerals. Peter and the doctor discussed whether feeling guilty and seeking justice was helpful for Peter's life and whether in reality he could have prevented any of the deaths. He discussed ways he could perform small personal rituals to 'say goodbye' but also ways he could honour the influence some of these people had had on his life and how he could carry their memories with him.

Over the next few weeks Peter realised there was no real evidence for what he had believed that his dead relatives thought of him. He began to feel stronger and to tell the doctor stories about how many of them had encouraged him and loved him. In particular he talked about his grandmother, who had 'grown him up', and about her wonderful sense of humour. The doctor gradually stopped his olanzepine, as she thought that the diagnosis of schizophrenia had been incorrect.

SOMATISATION AND SOMATOFORM DISORDER (MEDICALLY UNEXPLAINED SYMPTOMS)

The DSM-IV-TR describes somatoform disorders as 'the presence of physical symptoms that suggest a general medical condition and are not fully explained by a general medical condition, by the direct effects of a substance, or by another mental disorder. The symptoms must cause clinically significant distress or impairment in social, occupational, or other areas of functioning.'[8]

Somatisation (previously called hysteria) is a 'polysymptomatic disorder that begins before age 30 years, extends over a period of years, and is characterized by a combination of pain, gastrointestinal, sexual and pseudoneurological symptoms'.[8] This term has often come to be used in the same way that 'hysteria' was in the past, as a fairly derogatory description of someone who presents to health professionals constantly complaining of a collection of symptoms that have no physical basis.

Firstly, it must be remembered that many patients come from countries where serious diseases can present with vague symptoms in many different parts of the body. Tuberculosis, malaria, syphilis, HIV, strongyloides, hookworm, tapeworm and many other parasites and organisms are very common, particularly in developing countries. Patients who have come from cultures with limited mental health facilities or mental health literacy are more likely to suspect that their 'polysymptomatic disorder' is caused by a 'worm' rather than by a psychological problem. Research has shown neurobiological changes in patients complaining of 'somatisation', implying that even though a physical cause for their symptoms cannot be found, there are pathophysiological processes occurring that can explain some of the aspects of their illness.[9]

Using questions such as those in the Cultural Awareness Tool (Chapter 2) the health professional can quickly find out what the patient's symptoms mean to them, without having to use words or concepts that are unfamiliar to the patient. A discussion about how stress, worry, grief, sadness and other negative emotions can cause physical symptoms may be enough for the patient to take a different view of their illness and move away from their attachment to a physical cause. Such 'psychoeducation' will sometimes not change the patient's attitude immediately and several conversations may be needed before the patient understands to their satisfaction. They may need some help, such as behavioural techniques or CBT, to disentangle the physical symptoms and keep them from causing further anxiety or depression.

Some patients may still be unconvinced that there is not a physical cause for their problems. The health professional will then need to make a decision about which investigations they can justify financially and ethically to assist the patient in coming to a psychological diagnosis. It is important that both health professional and patient agree from the outset about which tests will be done and that this does not escalate into a cascade of more and more investigations to allay the patient's fears. A firm management plan with copies to both patient and health professional can be very helpful under these circumstances.

For some patients, education, time, investigations and support will still leave them with debilitating physical symptoms for which the health profession can find no cause and which the patient is convinced have a physical aetiology. It is important not to judge such people as hysterical, malingering or stupid. Just 30 years ago, multiple sclerosis and systemic lupus erythematosus were often treated as hysterical disorders of young women, purely because the medical profession had not yet developed investigations that confirmed the physical nature of these illnesses. Whatever the true cause of the symptoms, if the health profession cannot find a physical diagnosis or treatment, the patient must be assisted in overcoming their 'clinically significant distress or impairment in social, occupational, or other areas of functioning' as much as possible.[8] Techniques such as those used in narrative therapy (Chapter 5) can be very beneficial in this regard, as they separate the patient from the problem and can help them find a more meaningful life that is not controlled by their symptoms.

CONCLUSION

Many Western health professionals have a great deal of expertise in the use of cognitive behavioural therapy. With modifications their skills can be used across cultures but they will need to be aware of the innate ethnocentrism that is implicit in many of the techniques. Health professionals who are learning CBT, particularly those from collectivist cultures, may feel insecure about their ability to understand the cultural differences well enough to practise CBT. They may not be used to separating thoughts and feelings, be uncomfortable challenging patient's unconscious thoughts or unsure about their ability to help patients find solutions to problems that are outside their personal experience. Most of the behavioural techniques can be learnt and taught to patients no matter what the cultural background of the health professional. If the health professional has good insight into their own ethnocentricism, has good support, is flexible and is able to be honest with the patient, the other CBT techniques can similarly be modified so as to be useful across cultures.

Further reading

➤ Aisbett B. *Taming the Black Dog*. Sydney: HarperCollins; 2000.

➤ Burns D. *Feeling Good: the new mood therapy*. Sydney: HarperCollins; 1999.

➤ Howell C. *Keeping the Blues Away. A Guide to Managing Depression*. Adelaide: University of Adelaide; 2007. Available at: www.keepingthebluesaway.com

➤ Tanner S, Ball J. *Beating the Blues: a self-help approach to overcoming depression*. Sydney: Doubleday; 1989.

➤ Williams CJ. *Overcoming Depression: a five areas approach*. London: Arnold; 2001.

➤ Website – The Mood Gym – Delivering cognitive behavioural therapy for overcoming depression. Available at: www.moodgym.anu.edu.au/

REFERENCES

1 Moulding N, Hepworth J. Understanding body image disturbance in the promotion of mental health: a discourse analytic study. *J Community Appl Soc Psychol*. 2001; **11**: 305–17.

2 Mental Health Promotion and Illness Prevention. Auseinet. *Settings and Populations: mental health promotion and illness prevention – Aboriginal and Torres Strait Islander people*. Available at: www.auseinet.com/ppei/atsi.php (accessed April 2008).

3 Nyagua J, Harris A. West African refugee health in rural Australia: complex cultural factors that influence mental health. *Rural Remote Health*. 2008; **8**: 884. Available at: www.rrh.org.au/articles/subviewnew.asp?ArticleID=884 (accessed April 2008).

4 Abas M, Baingana F, Broadhead J, *et al*. Common mental disorders and primary health care: current practice in low-income countries. *Harv Rev Psychiatry*. 2003; **11**: 166–73.

5 Miller W, Rollnick S. *Motivational Interviewing: preparing people to change addictive behaviour*. New York: Guilford Press; 1991.

6 Prochaska JO, DiClemente CC, Norcross JC. In search of how people change. *Am Psychol*. 1992; **47**: 1102–4.

7 Andrews G. *Structured Problem Solving*. Available at: www.crufad.unsw.edu.au/phc/structuredproblemsolving.htm (accessed March 2008).

8 American Psychiatric Association. *Diagnostic and Statistical Manual of Mental Disorders: DSM-IV-TR*. 4th ed. Washington DC: APA; 1994.

9 Kirmayer L, Looper K. Abnormal illness behaviour: physiological, psychological and social dimensions of coping with distress. *Curr Opin Psychiatry*. 2006; **19**: 54–60.

5

Modified narrative therapy

This chapter explores:
- The concept of narrative therapy
- The importance of stories in constructing cultural identities
- The process of narrative therapy
- Dominant and alternative stories

Narrative therapy is an example of a 'patient-centred' psychotherapeutic technique. While many counselling techniques include stories or narratives as part of their process, the term narrative therapy specifically refers to a method devised by an Australian, Michael White, and a New Zealander, David Epston. The central tenet is that the patient never *is* or even *has* the problem but rather that the problem has come into the patient's life. As Michael White put it in the summer of 1988: 'The patient is not the problem, the problem is the problem.'[1] Patients are viewed as experts in their own lives and cultures, making it a patient-centred approach. However, while patient-centred consultations involve exploring a patient's ideas, concerns, expectations and the effects of the problem on his or her life, narrative therapy also looks at the effects of the patient's life on the problem. Thus, the main difference between the patient-centred therapies such as narrative therapy and cognitive behavioural therapy (CBT), for instance, is that narrative therapy explores the solution to the problem in detail rather than concentrating on the problem. It focuses on the patient's world and the life of the problem in that world. The therapist helps the patient use his or her own skills, beliefs, values, motivation and capabilities to help resolve the problem in the most appropriate way for that patient. Whereas CBT assumes that the patient's thoughts and actions are faulty and in need of repair, narrative therapy assumes that the patient is doing the best they can under the circumstances. In this chapter we look at the nature of narrative therapy and describe our modified approach to its use in transcultural interactions.

STORIES AND IDENTITY

Narrative therapy can be practised with only a minimal amount of knowledge of the other culture but involves a great deal of respect, genuine curiosity, active listening and reflective skills. Everyone has many different stories about their lives, past, present and future, which are all occurring simultaneously. Stories will be about aspects such as abilities, struggles, competencies, actions, desires, relationships, work, interests, conquests, achievements and failures.[2] Gender, sexuality, class, race, culture, family, community, power and religion all contribute to the identity each person builds up about themselves and their place in the world. As the stories are retold, certain events, skills and 'ways of being' are likely to be forgotten or ignored, depending on whether they fit in with the dominant plot.[2] In narrative therapy, the patient and the therapist together explore the stories about the patient's life and relationships, their effects, their meanings and their context. A summary of the foundations of narrative therapy is shown in Box 5.1.

BOX 5.1 NARRATIVE THERAPY

- Narrative therapy adopts a non-blaming approach.
- Patients are recognised as experts in their own lives.
- Problems are seen as separate from people.
- People have many skills, competencies, beliefs, values, commitments and abilities to help them change their relationship with problems in their lives.
- Patient and therapist must have curiosity and a willingness to ask questions to which the answers aren't obviously known.
- There are many possible directions that any therapeutic conversation can take.
- The patient plays a significant part in determining the directions that are taken.

Narrative therapy has been described as a postmodern approach which does not follow traditional psychological observations. Therapists believe that there are many different 'narratives' impacting on a person's life and that an individual is in a different position in each of them. There are numerous interpretations of a patient's stories and it is cultural and social factors, rather than biological and psychological factors, which help the patient make sense of experiences.[3] While narrative therapy has no set convention of length or timing of sessions, broadly speaking, therapy consists of working through a number of stages (Box 5.2).[3]

BOX 5.2 STAGES IN NARRATIVE THERAPY (ADAPTED FROM PAYNE[3])

- The patient tells their story, which includes an account of the problem(s).
- The therapist asks clarifying and extending questions, including effects of the problem on the patient's life.
- The patient is invited to give the problem a name – externalising the problem and acknowledging that it is having an effect on their life – it is external rather than internal or within the patient.
- Social, cultural and political issues are considered – is the patient blaming themself for any of these external and often power-based issues?
- Relative influence questioning – as well as considering the effect the problem has on the patient's life, they are asked to consider the effect they have on the life of the problem: when has the patient been able to manage or deal with this problem or similar ones?
- Exploring and magnifying an alternative story or 'marginalised narrative' – these are the parts of the narrative in which the patient has overcome the problem's influence.
- Enrichment of the 'unique outcomes' – building up a richer description of the circumstances in which the patient has overcome the problem.
- The patient is then invited to take a position on the problem – the patient can choose to remain in the existing narrative (dominant story) or take into account the narrative that the therapist has encouraged them to tell (alternative story).
- Continuing therapy – telling and re-telling the story.
- Ending therapy.

THE SCOPE OF NARRATIVE THERAPY

For patients from collectivist cultures such as the Australian Aboriginal people, narrative therapy allows the patient to find a story that gives them a sense of meaning and purpose in their lives that is likely to be different to that valued by the dominant culture. The Aboriginal Health Council of South Australia puts this quite succinctly:

In Western culture there is a dominant story about what it means to be a person of moral worth. This story emphasizes self-possession, self-containment, self-actualisation and so on. It stresses individuality at the expense of community and independence at the expense of connection. These are culturally specific values which are presented as universal, 'human' attributes to be striven for. The attempt to live up to these dominant prescriptions can have profoundly negative consequences for people's lives.[4]

People may be under pressure to conform to these 'normalising narratives'. Using narrative therapy, Aboriginal patients can reclaim their Aboriginal way of life with its emphasis on family responsibility, community, attachment to land, spirituality and traditional knowledge. They can strengthen this as their preferred story about their lives rather than that of the dominant culture. Authenticating spirituality and traditional therapies can have added benefits of assisting the healing process. This may need political and social action so that they can be sustained.

Similarly, many abused women, prisoners, people with HIV or with a disability may have internalised a story of failure, guilt or rejection about themselves determined by the surrounding dominant culture. Building up a new picture that affirms characteristics that may not be highly valued by the dominant culture will give them a sense of personal power and hope that acknowledges skills and resilience that are important in their subculture. As two narrative therapists wrote in 2002: 'By giving consideration to the politics involved in the shaping of identity, it becomes possible to enable new understandings of life that are influenced less by self-blame and more by an awareness of how our lives are shaped by broader cultural stories.'[5]

Narrative therapy can also bring cultural and community skills into the therapeutic encounter. It has been described as a 'way of bringing voices of our ancestors to therapeutic and community settings; honouring our cultural practices and traditions; reclaiming our particular ways of celebrating life; integrating spiritual elements that foster human connection and transformation; facilitating multicultural gatherings on the prevention of family violence . . . and exploring the importance of rituals, ceremonies, and stories of survival as sources of strength and unity'.[6]

People may present to a health professional complaining of a life that is saturated with problems. They feel that whatever coping mechanisms they have used in the past are no longer of benefit and they will often present in a crisis situation as the 'passive victim' of their troubles. Both patient and therapist may feel overwhelmed and helpless in the face of the difficulties of this 'problem-saturated story'. This is made more complex for the health professional if the patient comes from a culture that is different from their own, one with different beliefs, religion, views about health, education, morals, ethics or family and community expectations.

Patients with such illnesses as depression, anxiety, adjustment disorder and post-traumatic stress disorder (PTSD) and even those with schizophrenia have 'dominant stories' that they believe about themselves. However, there is always an 'alternative story', a different way of looking at this person's life, that will help them function more successfully as an individual, in their family and in their community. This is a way of working that takes into account the culture and history of a patient as well as the broader context that can affect people's lives.

THE PROCESS OF NARRATIVE THERAPY

(Definitions of common concepts in relation to narrative therapy are shown in Box 5.3.)

BOX 5.3 DEFINITIONS OF COMMON CONCEPTS

- Problem-saturated life – a life in crisis and overwhelmed with the problem.
- Dominant story – the story of the problem-saturated life.
- Externalising conversation – finding the nature of the problem and separating it from the person.
- Unique outcomes – those times when the problem has not 'won' dominance in the patient's life.
- Alternative story – the new story 're-authored' around the unique outcomes.

The first step in the process is to try to understand the patient, to listen carefully and respectfully to their story, all the time on the lookout for 'unique outcomes' that may be hidden in the narrative. This is one of the most difficult steps for health professionals who are usually trained to diagnose illness and to be 'problem-focussed' – to build up a picture of the patient's problem, find a solution or a treatment, present it to them, answer questions, organise review etc. In narrative therapy the health professional and patient build up a picture of the problem by 'externalising' it and look for times when the problem has been absent.

Having externalised the problem, the next step is to find out more about the effects the problem (the dominant story – Box 5.4) has on the patient's life. The health professional asks questions about how the problem 'learnt' to control the patient's life, who encourages or discourages it, what lies it is telling about the patient, what will happen if the problem continues to run the patient's life, when they are most vulnerable and what happens if the patient ignores the problem. Other questions can be asked that encourage the patient to map the influence of the problem in their lives. The health professional can then observe the problem's sphere of influence over the patient's behaviour, emotions, physical health, work, family life, relationships and attitude.[1] Skills can be explored that will assist the patient to escape or reclaim their life from the effects of the problem, revise their relationship with the problem or undermine the influence of the problem.[5]

BOX 5.4 THE DOMINANT STORY

- How did the problem come to be controlling your life?
- Who encourages it?
- Who discourages it?
- What lies does it tell you about yourself?
- How does it maintain its influence in your life?
- What happens if you ignore it?
- When is it most dangerous?
- Where are you most vulnerable to it taking control?

The coping mechanisms of the patient are multifactorial and will depend on such factors as their cultural background, childhood experiences, social circumstances, religion and of course the trigger for the current crisis. Whatever is happening at the time of the consultation, the patient has survived and coped up until that point. Narrative therapy attempts to access the patient's resilience, what skills they have used in the past, and even in the current circumstances, and what is happening when the problem is not 'winning' in the patient's life. The very fact that the patient has presented for help indicates that there are still some 'precious sparks of hope – the hope that things might be different at some future time'.[7] This glimmer of hope is often the only thing that has kept patients going through the problems that have overwhelmed them. The health professional will then assist the patient to build up those resources so that they are more able to deal with the current situation.

An alternative story (Box 5.5) develops based on the times when the patient has been successful rather than the problem, and this is then expanded into the present and then the future. Rather than develop an external 'observer ego' that examines the patient's life and problems from a distance, narrative therapy externalises the problem and locates the patient's successful characteristics and stories within. The family and community can then unite with the patient and the therapist as they all stand together to help develop solutions to the power the problem has over the patient's life. The patient is not the 'outsider'; the problem is the 'outsider'. Building up a 'rich description' of the alternative story and its possibilities gives the patients more options for change in their lives. It enables the patient to see that their life is not just about problems and difficulties, but that it is also about 'hopes, dreams, passions, principles, achievements, skills, abilities and more'.[5] A good sense of humour is a huge advantage in narrative therapy. By laughing with the patient during the process of externalising the problem, the health professional and the patient are already working together to decrease its power.

The Chinese pictogram that makes up the word 'crisis' has two characters – danger and opportunity. The health professional's job is to help the patient to move the crisis situation from one of 'danger' to one of 'opportunity'. To do this they must listen carefully for evidence of resilience in the past, 'unique outcomes' in the present and 'precious sparks of hope' when discussing the future. They might be curious about when the patient was last feeling happy or successful, and pay close attention to subtle changes in body language when telling different stories about the present. When evidence of resilience, a unique outcome or hope is discovered, the health professional can then ask questions that will develop a better picture of the circumstances surrounding the alternative story. They can ask 'who, what, when, where, how . . .?' not about the problem, but about the resilience, unique outcome or hope.

BOX 5.5 THE ALTERNATIVE STORY

- Can you think of a time when the problem did not control your life?
- Who can encourage you to build up the alternative story?
- What would that person tell me about you?
- What else can you do to decrease the problem's control over your life?
- What can you say to yourself to challenge the problem's lies?
- Do you need to find some distractions from the problem's strong messages?
- What would life look like if the problem did not control your life so much?

Narrative therapy is very useful in some patients with severe PTSD, such as people who have been refugees. The fear, rage and guilt cycle may have eroded any respect they have for themselves by the time the health professional gets to see them, and often their relationship with their spouse and children is also very tenuous. They certainly feel saturated with the problem and out of control of their own lives, with a huge burden of hopelessness and despair. Most have suffered enormous hardship to settle in countries such as Australia and then have to grapple with a very different way of life. To externalise the PTSD and revisit characteristics such as courage, loyalty, patience, creative thinking, intelligence and love can help them re-establish self-respect for themselves as being a worthwhile person. Presenting this alternative view to the family can also help them develop ways to break the cycle and start again to behave with courage and love.

BOX 5.6 CASE STUDY 1 (RAZZAQ'S STORY)

Razzaq came to Australia as a refugee from Iraq. After escaping Saddam Hussein's regime and a hair-raising trip in an overcrowded boat, he was held in a detention centre for two years. He was then given a temporary visa for another three years, suffering constant fear that he would be sent back to Iraq. Finally, he received a permanent visa, and recently his wife and family have joined him in Australia.

Razzaq has times when he suddenly becomes very afraid when something quite minor happens like his wife turns on the washing machine without telling him or he hears a car backfire in the distance. It reminds him of some of the noises from the war. He gets very angry and often yells at his wife and has even hit her once or twice. Sometimes he also yells at the children for very minor things. He feels very guilty then and tells himself that he is a bad husband and father. He often convinces himself that they would be better off without him because of these unpredictable attacks and then hides away for days because of the guilt. He only sleeps a few hours a night because of the awful nightmares.

The doctor listened to the story and then asked if there is anyone who disagrees with this view he has about himself. Razzaq told a story about someone he met the other day who knew him before the war. They talked about what a good journalist he had been and how difficult it was when your brain didn't work like it used to because of all the awful pictures in it. The friend congratulated him on getting himself and his whole family out of the country safely and said what a good father and husband he must be. He came home and told his wife about the friend and she cried and said that he was a good husband and father and this madness would never take that away.

The doctor encouraged this view of himself as being the 'real' Razzaq. They discussed how the PTSD had clouded this picture and how guilt, depression and social isolation were making it worse. They also discussed how strong his love was for his family, as he was so upset and guilty when he hurt them. Razzaq's wife was asked to join the consultation and the three began building a new picture of how Razzaq could distract himself from the anger with such things as exercise and music, how the triggers in the household could be decreased, how socialising with people who knew this 'real' Razzaq would help him to be stronger and how he needed constantly to remind himself about his love, courage and perseverance. With his wife's help he was able to forgive himself when he had an angry outburst or found it impossible to concentrate, and he began to feel safer to play and laugh with his children.

BOX 5.7 CASE STUDY 2 (STEVEN'S STORY)

Steven is 32 and was recently diagnosed with HIV as part of the screening process before being accepted into university to start a dentistry degree. He was shocked to hear of the diagnosis, as he has never used drugs and has not had a sexual partner for the last five years. After talking to the doctor he realised that he probably contracted the disease in his early 20s when he had a few brief relationships with other men and didn't use protection. He is unable to start the dentistry course even though he has quit his IT job to begin university. He told the doctor he feels like a leper and that if people find out he has HIV, they won't want to know him. They'll think he is promiscuous and stupid and will be afraid to even talk to him, let alone touch him. He says he feels stupid for catching HIV and he can never forgive himself for getting it. He thinks it has ruined his life and that he has no friends, will never get a good job, will be sick for the rest of his life and will probably die soon anyway.

The doctor talked to Steven about how HIV is not the whole story about his life and that most of his personality and skills are still the same. As part of trying to help him to socialise again she suggested he join a support group for people with HIV. Steven has had to come to terms with his own judgemental attitude toward people with HIV, that they 'should have known better', and has realised that most of the other people in the group are struggling with the same issues as he is. Members of the group realised that there are quite a few of them that are musical and they recently played at a gathering to raise money for the AIDS Council. Many people came up afterwards and congratulated them. Steven was talking to someone from a medical technology company who was very interested in his IT skills. He asked if Steven would like to come and do some casual work while another employee was away for six months. He was surprised that even though this man knew he had HIV, he still wanted to employ him.

In trying to help Steven with his depression and isolation, the doctor talked about the 'unique outcomes' of the HIV support group and the new IT position. Steven spoke about how in externalising the HIV he was able to see that he could have friends, social support and maybe even a new career.

PRACTICAL POINTS

➤ The Dulwich Centre website is a very useful source of information on narrative therapy: www.dulwichcentre.com.au
➤ Narrative therapy is a patient-centred approach that is problem-focussed but also concentrates on exploring the solution to the problem.
➤ Narrative therapy is a useful approach in transcultural consultations.
➤ The health professionals must demonstrate a great deal of respect, genuine curiosity, active listening and reflective skills.

REFERENCES

1 White M. The externalizing of the problem and the re-authoring of lives and relationships. *Dulwich Centre Newsletter*. Adelaide: Dulwich Centre Publications; summer 1988–89.
2 Morgan A. *What is Narrative Therapy? An Easy to Read Introduction*. Dulwich: Dulwich Centre Publications; 2000. Available at: www.dulwichcentre.com.au/alicearticle.html (accessed March 2008).
3 Payne M. *Narrative Therapy*. 2nd ed. London: Sage; 2006.
4 Aboriginal Health Council of South Australia. Reclaiming our stories, reclaiming our lives: an initiative of the Aboriginal Health Council of South Australia. *Dulwich Centre Newsletter*. 1995; 1: 1–40.
5 Carey M, Russell S. *Externalising Commonly Asked Questions*. 2002. Available at: www. dulwichcentre.com.au/externalising.htm (accessed April 2008).
6 Rojas R, Montgomery P, Tovar J. Reflections on language, power, culture and spirituality: our experience of the conference. *Narrative Therapy and Community Work: a conference collection*. Adelaide: Dulwich Centre Publications; 1999.
7 White M. *Re-authoring Lives: interviews and essays*. Adelaide: Dulwich Centre Publications; 1995.

6

Resilience and spirituality

This chapter explores:
- The concepts of resilience and spirituality in the management of mental health problems across all cultures
- How the concepts may be applied in a practical sense in the care of patients

> In the midst of a turbulent, often chaotic life we are called to reach out, with courageous honesty to our innermost self, with relentless care to our fellow human beings and with increasing prayer to our God.
>
> *Henri JM Nouwen*[1]

Resilience may be conceptualised as reflecting the positive capacity of a person to bounce back from adverse events such as conflict or failure, and to learn from positive events such as increased responsibility; it is a dynamic process rather than a static state or an attribute.[2]

PROTECTIVE AND RISK FACTORS IN MENTAL HEALTH

Resilience is about transforming the adversity that comes into all our lives into 'wisdom, insight and compassion' (p. 6).[3] The World Health Organization defines health as a state of 'complete physical, mental and social well-being' and goes on to say that 'mental health can be conceptualized as a state of well-being in which the individual realizes his or her own abilities, can cope with the normal stresses of life, can work productively and fruitfully, and is able to make a contribution to his or her community.'[4] The National Aboriginal Community Controlled Health Organisation defines health as 'not just the physical wellbeing of an individual, but the social, emotional, and cultural wellbeing of the whole community in which each individual is able to achieve their full potential as a human being thereby bringing about the total wellbeing of their community'.[5] Resilience and an individual's ability to 'bounce back' and learn from hardship in order to reach their potential are pivotal to mental health.

Psychological problems will start to develop in anyone when the stresses they are encountering are beyond their personal resources. Some of the factors that are protective against mental dysfunction tend to be universal but different cultures, religions, societies, families and individuals will value these protective factors to varying degrees (Box 6.1). Those who come from a culture that tends to promote 'resilience-producing' characteristics are likely to be able to cope with more stressful circumstances and to recover from challenging times (for example, *see* Box 6.2 below). Stressors at a socioenvironmental level and the individual's ability to deal with these at a personal and community level are directly linked to the aetiology of most mental disorders.[6] Resources and supports will also be evident to a different extent. Supportive society structures, efficient personal communication styles, effective community leaders and flexible systems of belief will all aid in resilience. Different cultures will encourage certain personality styles such as hardiness, ego strength, a sense of coherence, optimism and humour.[7] Children will be protected from danger and hardship and nurtured differently. They will be expected to 'stand on their own two feet' at different ages.

BOX 6.1 FACTORS AFFECTING RESILIENCE AND MENTAL HEALTH

- Childhood history (especially relationship with mother).
- Genetic predisposition.
- Personality.
- Finances.
- Education.
- Health (including diet, exercise, self-care).
- Spirituality.
- Religion (rules and rituals).
- Sense of humour.
- Supportive relationships.
- Locus of control.
- Personal insight.

BOX 6.2 CASE STUDY 1 ON RESILIENCE (ALIMAMY'S STORY)

Alimamy came to see the doctor soon after her arrival in her new country from a refugee camp in West Africa. She was the wife of a chief who had found himself at odds with the government in power. They raided the house, stabbed him to death, raped their 13-year-old daughter to death and then burnt the house with the bodies in it. They raped Alimamy and tied her up. She was eight and a half months pregnant. They then heard gunshots in the distance and ran away. Her five-year-old twin daughters untied her and they fled with her young son through the forest. No one would take them in, as everyone was afraid of having the same thing done to them. On arrival a week later at the border they were thrown into prison until United Nations personnel found them and took them to a refugee camp.

When Alimamy first arrived in her new country she was very anxious and was having nightmares and flashbacks of what had happened. She had not had any medical care in the camp over the previous three years and had not told anyone what had really happened to her. Gradually she told her story, received appropriate medical care and became well. One day she told the doctor she now wanted to start to train as a nurse so that she could help people again.

The doctor asked her how it was that she was able to deal with all this so well. She said 'I am a chief's wife and by the grace of God I am a woman of great courage and wisdom.' Her resilience was something that was an integral part of her personality; she would always be a chief's wife.

There are those who manage to maintain their hope, a sense of humour, a deep spirituality, their ability to creatively problem-solve and a meaning and purpose in life, despite the other parameters being stacked up against them. However, patients with mental illness who come to see health professionals may have very few of these factors to draw upon. Many of the psychotherapies in use today aim to improve insight, an internal locus of control and relationships and to encourage education, deeper spirituality, better self-care and a sense of humour. Religion may be a source of guilt and stress or a source of comfort. Health professionals can encourage patients to seek religious counselling if they see this as an important part of the patient's management plan.

RESILIENCE AND MENTAL HEALTH

Many of the factors that affect resilience will differ from culture to culture. Lack of education for girls, the 'normalisation' of domestic violence and incest in some cultures, early arranged marriage, religious traditions, gender differences, access to healthcare, war, poverty, inequality – these appear to be immutable. Settling into a new country will be difficult whether the person has come as a refugee, a skilled migrant, a student or an international medical graduate. The 'culture shock' of landing in a different climate with different food, different language, different clothes and different social and cultural rules will obviously have an effect on resilience in the short term.

In looking at different societies that have been through extreme trauma, there are some groups who consistently seem to maintain their resilience. There are others who fall into despair and become the 'passive victims' to their circumstances. This is not a genetic or racial characteristic. Resilience is learnt, 'hard-wired' into the brains of children so they learn that there are some people who are trustworthy, develop a set of beliefs that guide how they respond to the world and feel that they are loved and are capable of love and respect. These character traits then become the unconscious coping patterns that they carry through life. Resilience becomes their 'normal' behaviour. This is likely to be more common in collectivist cultures as well as those families, societies and cultures that value children and nurture close and loving relationships.

THE GENETICS OF RESILIENCE

Medicine has long known that there is a genetic predisposition to most mental illnesses but there is emerging evidence that there are also 'resilience genes' that protect some people from becoming depressed under extreme stress. Research has mostly been done on the 5-HTTLPR variation and genes that carry the code for the serotonin transporter protein. The 5-HTT allele can be either long or short. Those people with two long alleles have a better chance of bouncing back after adverse life events. Those who have one short allele will have less resilience and those with two short, a greater chance of depression. However, it's only under extreme circumstances such as child abuse, war or chronic stress that the gene will be 'triggered'. Those people who do not experience severe life events will not have an increased rate of depression if they have the short allele. The other important finding is that there is a protective effect of good social supports that can counteract both the genetic and the environmental risk.[8]

RESILIENCE AND SOCIAL DETERMINANTS OF WELL-BEING

Many people from indigenous cultures and developing countries live in poverty without adequate housing, education or healthcare needs being met. Helping them to gain a sense of meaning and purpose in their lives is best done in conjunction with addressing the social determinants of health that are affecting their psychological well-being. Even the most skilled psychotherapist will find it much harder to be helpful if the patient is hungry and there are 14 people living in a two-bedroom house.

Those who suffer from extreme poverty and who are victims of torture or trauma are unlikely to have gained a sense of resilience even if their family environment is stable and loving. Assaults on the brain development of children such as malnutrition, severe illness, sexual abuse and experiencing extremely traumatic events are likely to leave long-lasting scars. These children are unlikely to grow up feeling that the world is a safe place, that relationships are nurturing and that there is hope for the future. Helping these adults become mentally healthy will need long-term treatment, as new connections need to develop in their brains to replace those that have developed in their childhood.

BOX 6.3 CASE STUDY 2 (FATIMA AND MARIAM'S STORIES)

Fatima and Mariam are both refugees who have recently arrived from the Middle East to reunite with their husbands. The men have been in detention in Australia for about five years and still struggle with post-traumatic stress disorder (PTSD). The wives come with several children and both became pregnant soon after arrival.

Both of these women are illiterate and speak no English. They were both married at the age of 13 and both have an older daughter who helps them with housework, shopping etc. Besides their children and husbands, neither have any other relatives in Australia.

Fatima is extremely depressed and demanding. She regularly misses appointments, often comes to the surgery complaining of pain, fatigue and insomnia having taken none of the medication suggested at the previous appointment and is prone to outbursts of crying and rage. She has no friends and relies on her 15-year-old daughter for physical and emotional support. She and her husband are constantly arguing and she is always very angry with him. She does not have much of a spiritual faith, does not have a good relationship with her own mother or siblings, has no real interests or hobbies, does not exercise and often relates as though she is still aged 13.

Mariam on the other hand is full of life and fun. She is very excited to be back with her husband, as he is with her. They are cousins and have grown up in a very supportive and caring extended family. Many of their beloved relatives are in various countries throughout the world and they continue to have as much contact as possible. She encourages her children to go to school, as she wants them to have opportunities she didn't have. She has joined an English class and has a fulfilling and meaningful spiritual life, especially now she is reunited with her husband.

With very similar cultural backgrounds these two women cope very differently with their new lives. Growing up in a caring family, good current support, a sense of humour, outside interests, a meaningful faith and an altruistic outlook all contribute to Mariam's resilience.

When trying to help Fatima, a health professional will need to acknowledge that her difficulties stem from more than just her culture and her current circumstances. Helping Fatima find resources within herself will be difficult, as she has very few factors in her life to give her resilience.

Many Western cultures have neglected to prioritise connections with family, including laughter, and spiritual and moral values for children. The individualism and materialism that are the hallmarks of Western culture behave like a 'cultural antagonist' to many of the aspects of spirituality, making it almost impossible to acknowledge the importance of other people and community.[9] As Western countries become richer there has been an increase in television and computer use, a quest for individual achievement in sport and academia and a decrease in the time children spend with parents and extended families. The increase in riches has not seen an increase in happiness. It certainly hasn't seen an increase in resilience and is often blamed for a perceived increase in irresponsibility and lack of 'community spirit' in many young people.

Many see pain, suffering, mistakes and 'failure' as abnormal parts of life that should not happen. They look to blame someone or something and do not look for the opportunity for renewal and learning that comes from the experience. For those who have grown up in a culture where individual effort, economic success and competitiveness are valued, failure may not be seen as an inevitable part of life that leads to creativity and learning but as a cause for guilt that they have done a terrible thing. Others feel overwhelming shame and hide or run away rather than try to repair mistakes or heal damaged relationships.[10]

Without a sense of community, of caring for each other, of purpose that is beyond individual effort, of being connected to others no matter what has happened and of sharing hardship, many people lose hope. The rise in suicide rates throughout the world and the enormous 'business' of psychotherapy and psychopharmacology is evidence that Western culture is not serving its followers well as far as mental health goes.

There is a small wave of groups, teachers, health professionals and even politicians who have realised the importance of teaching children skills in resilience from birth and of encouraging early relationships with parents and other caring individuals and communities. Programmes to teach parents, children and young adults how to encourage resilience are springing up and new disciplines such as early childhood and infant mental health acknowledge that nurturing psychological well-being and skills are important as early as possible.

LEARNING AND TEACHING RESILIENCE

Much of today's psychotherapy aims to teach skills that resilient people have learnt in childhood. Problem solving, balance, self-care, insight, realistic expectations, relationship skills, compassion, living in the present, asking for help, facing mistakes, seeing the bigger picture – these are the lessons modern patients are learning from psychotherapists rather than from families, culture and society. Health professionals are the ones who are assisting patients in coming to see that there is greater purpose in life that surpasses their own individual effort and that what they do is important to other people and their community.

For those who have shown resilience in the past but have become besieged by hardship and have temporarily lost hope and meaning, the aim of psychotherapy is likely to be different. They are more likely to have a support system in place, to feel connected to other people and to have spiritual beliefs and religious practices that have sustained them in the past. They may need help with something like housing or finances. They may need help accessing their own problem-solving ability or to be reminded of their courage and wisdom in the past. They may also need help in finding spiritual nourishment in a strange environment. But they may just need to have a health professional listen to their story with respect and empathy.

SPIRITUALITY

Spirituality and religious practices are both important features of a person's resilience. Particularly at times of stress and illness people are likely to question their purpose in life, their relationship with the world and with God and the meaning of suffering and death. The health profession currently seems to be moving into the 'age of empowerment' where patient dignity is more likely to be maintained and interventions to be more appropriate.[11] In a multicultural society this will need to take into account a patient's religious and spiritual beliefs and resources.

Spirituality can be defined as 'the ways in which people fulfil what they consider to be the purpose of their lives, through finding hope or inner peace'.[9] For many, spirituality will be expressed in the religious practices of their cultural upbringing or their individual preference. For others, spirituality will be a relationship with a 'higher being' or 'the universe' or may be more secular in its expression. Still others will find it through music, art or a connection with the environment.

Richard Eckersley brings together culture, spirituality and religion when he says:

> Cultures are about how we think the world 'works': the language, knowledge, beliefs, assumptions and values that shape how we see the world and our place in it; give meaning to our experience; and are passed between individuals, groups and generations. Spirituality is a deeply intuitive, but not always consciously expressed, sense of connectedness to the world in which we live. Its most common cultural representation is religion, an institutionalised system of belief and ritual worship that usually centres on a supernatural god or gods.[9]

Health professionals and patients moving to Westernised countries may notice a lack of religious observance within the population. Many people from Western countries may not appear to be as religious, as these societies do not tend to integrate religion into everyday life as much as it is in some countries. In the West, religion has come to be part of an individual's private life rather than an established part of society or culture. Moreover, in multicultural societies many religions co-exist, alongside the ideas of agnosticism and atheism. Usually there is tolerance and compromise in such societies, but obviously religious tension may occur. A more dominant religion in a multicultural society may be judgemental or discriminatory against those who follow other religions, sometimes with the support of the government.

HEALTH AND HOLISTIC CARE

Western medicine works mainly within the biomedical model of illness causation. This approach is limited because it does not take into account that health and illness are also shaped by personal, psychological, spiritual and social as well as biological factors. The model leads to a disease-centred approach, where the main tasks of the doctor are to diagnose illness from a biological perspective and to treat it, hopefully effecting a cure. The drive to make an 'evidence-based' diagnosis is extremely strong. The biomedical model disconnects medicine from the social and spiritual fabric of patients' lives.[12]

The biopsychosocial model is an improvement on this reductionist approach. This recognises that a patient's problem may be defined in terms of its physical, psychological and social components (the biopsychosocial model[13,14]). Health professionals are usually trained to be objective and not to impose their belief systems onto the patient, but in so doing may also be keeping the patient's spiritual beliefs, resources and practices out of the consultation.[9] Religious beliefs can merely be a part of a person's culture, be based more on rules and ritual or be about a spiritual relationship with a higher being.

If we consider the four dimensions of patient-centred care as physical, psychological, social and spiritual, we are moving towards holistic care. Health professionals who do not consider themselves as 'religious' may not think to make inquiries of patients in this domain. When working across cultures, health professionals may often come into contact with deeply held spiritual and religious beliefs that may not be those of the practitioner. Therapists may shy away from treading on this 'holy ground' for fear of offending patients but in so doing may have little access to either a causative factor of psychological distress or to a source of relief from that distress.

On the other hand, patients who do not identify themselves as religious or belonging to a particular religion may find it uncomfortable to be asked about such matters by health professionals who feel that religious observance is an important component of a person's life.

THE HIERARCHY OF HUMAN NEEDS

Maslow's hierarchy of human needs[15] (Figure 6.1) highlights the importance of survival, safety, love and belongingness before the 'higher levels' can be reached. For many people throughout the world, life is an everyday struggle with little hope of much more. Some would see that mystical or 'transcendent' spirituality is only possible at the highest level. 'Sociocentric' cultures may not view the concept of the 'actualisation' of self as the pinnacle of maturity and certainly not see it as necessary to reach the 'peak' of spirituality. Without doubt a strong spiritual faith has sustained many people through hardships when those people have been struggling for their everyday survival. Deep spiritual connectedness and meaning can transcend personal circumstances, social situations and what is happening in everyday life.[8] The observance of religious rituals themselves can also be important for some people and can help them cope with illness and distress even when spiritual faith is lacking or doubt has taken over.

The hierarchy of human needs alerts therapists to the importance of a holistic view of emotional and spiritual health. A truly healthy person – physically, psychologically and spiritually – is likely to have the needs of the whole pyramid met. A person's full potential for psychological and spiritual well-being may not be able to be reached if his or her physiological or safety needs have not been met. Many people will be capable of functioning at a 'higher level', including having a deep and enriching spiritual life, but may not be able to sustain this, as the other needs will become a priority at some point.

The mysteries and 'miracles' of how the mind works are often thought to be the work of a supernatural power. Even in Western culture, therapists such as Carl Jung discussed concepts such as the 'collective unconscious' using spiritual imagery and often overt spiritual references.

CONSIDERING RELIGIOUS BELIEFS

Attitudes to religion can be broadly divided into certain categories. Each category can have both negative and positive effects on a person's well-being, particularly on their mental health, depending on how they view God and

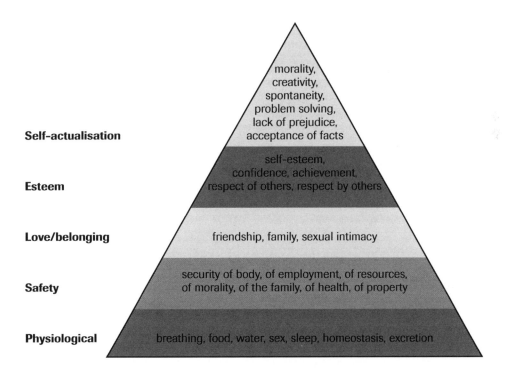

FIGURE 6.1 Maslow's hierarchy of human needs[15]

the world. A health professional may be able to guide a patient to take a more positive view of their relationship with God and the world, without necessarily changing their general opinion about their religion, if it seems that their outlook is detrimental to their health. Similarly, religious communities can either be supportive and give wise guidance and encouragement or be judgemental, restrictive and even dangerous.

1 A belief that God is all-knowing and all-seeing and that there are a set of rules to live by

If this belief is strongly held as the main view of God, the patient may feel paranoid, judged and anxious. They may fear that they are never able to please God and so become a perfectionist who is always depressed as they are unable to reach the goal of perfection. Despite striving to follow the rules set out by their religion they may always feel deficient and liable to be punished. The religious group may encourage this view if they feel that religious observances are directly linked to a person's health. If a patient does not become well, they may say that it's because they have not prayed enough, given enough money or paid enough obeisance to the appropriate deity.

On the other hand, those who believe in a more benevolent view of God may find it a comfort that they can live life knowing that they are unable to lie to God and that he/she still cares for them. They see the rules as guidelines for a better life and strive to follow them to the best of their ability. Taking part in religious rituals may be seen as part of the relationship with God, which can lead people closer to God because they are pleasing him/her. This can lead to a feeling of being supported and less isolated.

2 A belief that God is within each of us

Those who hold this belief may seem to others to be acting as though they themselves are God. They may have a strong sense of their own 'rightness', with a self-entitled, opinionated, sometimes narcissistic view of themselves. This may make them charismatic and attractive but may also lead to problems in their relationships and community. They are unlikely to have any insight into a negative side of themselves and be difficult to engage in any form of psychotherapy.

The other side of this belief may be that people see that everyone is a 'child of God' with the potential to do good. This may engender forgiveness, respect and benevolence both in how they relate to themselves and to others, even if they have harmed them or are their enemies. They may guide their actions by asking themselves – 'What would a loving God do in this situation both for myself and for the other person?'

3 A belief that God is primarily interested in justice and fairness

Sayings such as 'Do unto others as you would have them do unto you', 'Good things happen to good people and bad things happen to bad people', 'You get what you deserve' and 'What goes around comes around' have crept into the English vernacular because of this belief. Such convictions can lead people to perform 'good works' in the hope that good things will come to them in return but when 'bad' things happen they are likely to see this as a punishment for things they have done. This fatalism is very difficult to challenge.

For others the concept that our definition of 'justice and fairness' may be different from God's can guide this belief. Often people may trust that they may not be able to see immediate 'justice and fairness', particularly for themselves, but that in the long-term God has their interests at heart. For some this will be about lessons learnt and wisdom gained, for others the 'justice' or lessons may not come in this life but after this life has ended. This belief can also help explain many of life's difficulties by trusting the 'will of God'. As well as traditional Christian beliefs, the Islamic 'inshallah', the Chinese 'wu-wei' and the Hindu and Buddhist idea of 'kharma' can be invoked to free an individual from personal responsibility and leave life's circumstances and difficulties to a higher power.

4 A mystical belief

Mystics in any religion are often seen as being on a 'higher plane' than regular human beings. They may spend their time 'liaising with God', meditating or taking part in complex rituals. This may be quite an impractical way of life if they do not have the support of a dedicated community, as activities of daily living such as eating, washing and earning a living may suffer and relationships may not be nurtured. The burden and loneliness of being an 'elder' in a community may leave them very psychologically vulnerable.

A true mystic may have a relationship with God that gives them wisdom balanced with a sense of humility that is beyond usual human understanding. This may nourish them through many difficulties, and their resilience and quiet authority may also be a strength to others. They may be comfortable discussing their own behaviour, with an insight that does not carry any shame or fear, as they are confident about their relationship with God.

BOX 6.4 CASE STUDY 3 (KAMIZ'S STORY)

Kamiz had been a journalist in Iraq who had been imprisoned and very badly tortured. He had severe post-traumatic stress disorder (PTSD) and found it impossible to sit in the doctor's windowless office for more than about 10 minutes. He would become visibly distressed, shaky and sweaty and would startle at the sound of every footstep in the corridor. Medication and attempts at informal psychotherapy outside at the coffee shop down the road had made no real impact on his flashbacks, insomnia, panic attacks or other symptoms. One hot year in Ramadan he strode confidently into the doctor's office, greeted her warmly and sat down and smiled. The doctor was quite taken aback and expressed surprise at someone looking so cheerful during the month of fasting when most people were struggling to get through the day and did not leave the house because of the weather. Kamiz said that he was feeling fantastic as he had decided to continue smoking this Ramadan. The doctor chastised him good-naturedly as this is usually forbidden and he was a very religious man. Kamiz said that Allah was benevolent and understanding and had his best interests at heart. He was smoking because he *could* – no one was going to arrest him, spit on him, beat him or turn him in to the authorities. He was a free man in Australia and could have his own relationship with Allah, not one that was dictated to him by the government. He said that Allah would forgive him and that he would stop smoking again for Ramadan next year as was his usual practice. Kamiz had only minimal symptoms of PTSD from that time on. His relationship with God was extremely important and he was able to separate the inflexibility of the 'rules' of his religion so as to deepen that relationship, improve his sense of himself as a valuable human being and to heal.

DEFINING SPIRITUALITY

For many clerics and believers throughout the world their religion is the only true one and they aim to protect it from the influence of 'heretics' and secular society. However, spirituality is not necessarily synonymous with religion. Only 30% of Australians who value spirituality attend a religious service at least every month.[16]

Definitions of spirituality stress the concept's sense of meaning and purpose in life. People feel they belong – though whom they belong to varies. Spirituality encompasses wholeness and integration, harmony with the world, belief in the infinite and life being a journey towards attainment. People who do not believe in God and therefore do not fit within established religious practice may be spiritual and feel a sense of connection with the universe. Spirituality may be felt in different ways by different people but its importance to mental health and mental healing is increasingly being recognised within mainstream medicine, especially psychiatry. Box 6.5 lists some of the benefits for patients of interacting with the spiritual dimension.

BOX 6.5 BENEFITS OF SPIRITUALITY[17]

- Improved self-control.
- Improved self-esteem and confidence.
- Healthy grieving of loss through recognition of its normality.
- Improved relationships with self, others and creation (and/or God).
- A new sense of meaning.
- Renewed hope and peace of mind.
- Acceptance of things that cannot be changed.

In most cultures the unconscious and the spirit are seen as very closely connected. There seems to be some measure of yearning for a spiritual life in most people but how this is expressed as religion depends on cultural upbringing and individual choice. Creative pursuits such as music, art and dance are often part of religious observances but may also be a path to spirituality for many people who do not hold traditional religious beliefs. Similarly, an appreciation of nature and the importance of the environment are strong features in some religions but for others who do not believe in a particular religion they can guide them towards a deeper appreciation of the meaning of life and its connections. Whatever the religion, and whether people ascribe to a religion or not, the more spiritual people are, the more likely they are to have more similarities than differences.

Followers of most of the world's religions will range from the nominal to the fundamentalist and from the conservative to the mystical. Knowing the basic tenets of a religion will certainly help, but stereotyping people will not be of use for the patient or the mental health practitioner.

NEW AGE MYSTICISM

While health professionals are able for the most part to work with people with belief in one of the established religions, and indeed may follow one of these themselves, they may find it more difficult to interact with patients who have adopted a 'New Age' approach to life. New Age is a misnomer, as this spiritual lifestyle derives much of its ethos from Eastern religions and philosophy, though it may also be integrated with pagan and other Western old faiths. People who identify with New Age beliefs often come into conflict with their scientific evidence-based health providers. The New Age adherent is likely to decline immunisation and turn to complementary therapies for managing disease. They may seek advice from orthodox doctors but then decide to disregard their advice, causing ill-feeling between doctor and patient.

The logical mind of the university-trained physician will probably fail to see the potential in crystal healing, iridology and chanting, though he or she may be happy to recommend acupuncture and even meditation.

BOX 6.6 MICHAEL MCKNIGHT AT THE CRYSTAL BALL[18]

'Metaphysically, the quartz crystal can be easily programmed to help provide a positive outcome. It can clear away negative energy from the aura and re-align the chakra (energy) centers of the body. It can be useful in long distance healing through imaging and meditation . . . OK, OK, but how do they actually work??

Fact is I don't really know, but it must have something to do with faith, believing, imaging, and the greater god consciousness that is beyond words or speech. I know that there are nice folks out there in the world that would never believe that a rock or such could ever help them in any way. If it is true that we actually live many many lives and reincarnation is fact, then these people are simply in a particular incarnation that precludes them from having such beliefs (this time around).'

New Age is usually thought to have begun in the late 1960s with the hippie generation. Free love, helped by the introduction of the oral contraceptive pill, and mind-enhancing/expanding drugs were a feature of the movement. The traditional religions of their parents were no longer relevant to this younger generation, who looked for other meanings to life and who espoused peace and harmony. The Beatles increased the interest in meditation, and yoga also became popular. This way of life still exists, though it has changed over the years. One of the main hallmarks is a dislike of Western medicine and a desire to use 'natural' remedies rather than man-made chemicals (though of course all plants ultimately consist of chemicals). The modern New Age disciple will usually not wish to take antidepressants but would be open to appropriate counselling or psychotherapy that recognised the spiritual side of the problem.

BOX 6.7 CASE STUDY 4 (JOHN'S STORY)

John P was a 45-year-old decorator who lived with his wife, a trained counsellor. Both of them preferred natural and alternative therapies to prescribed drugs. John became depressed and decided to he see his GP. John had insight into his low mood and felt that he couldn't work while he was feeling so bad. He had no thoughts of self-harm and mainly wanted a medical certificate. He said his wife had recommended he see a counsellor friend of hers and also to have crystal therapy. The GP advised him to seek help from one person at a time, rather than overload himself with different opinions and treatments, however 'natural' they seemed, and to return for follow-up the next week. John did not come back until a fortnight had passed. The GP was concerned as he was obviously a lot worse – he looked dishevelled and tired. John said he had seen the counsellor, the crystal therapist and also a faith healer and naturopath. Each therapist had suggested a different root cause for his problems and a different type of treatment. John was extremely confused and was blaming himself for his symptoms. He had also spent a lot of money. He was having suicidal ideas. Eventually he agreed to see a perceptive and sympathetic psychiatrist, who started him on medication and helped him to explore the impact of the depression on his life and relationship.

John's story illustrates the idea that New Age therapy does not always sit well with orthodox medicine but that compromises may be made on both sides so that the patient's choice of therapy becomes truly complementary to the doctor's choice. The patient and doctor work in partnership and discuss the advantages and disadvantages of possible treatments, with the doctor accepting that the patient's beliefs, including spiritual ones, are valid.

SPIRITUALITY IN THE CONSULTATION

Any health professional can ask simple questions as suggested by the American College of Physicians such as:[19]
- ➤ is faith (religion, spirituality) important to you?
- ➤ has faith (religion, spirituality) been important to you at other times in your life?
- ➤ do you have someone to talk to about religious matters?
- ➤ would you like to explore religious or spiritual matters with someone?

In helping patients deal with spiritual issues as part of their psychological health, it is useful to know more about how their spirituality fits into the rest of their life, how important religion is in their spirituality, their attitudes to their religious beliefs, and how they express their spirituality (as compared to their religion). All of this can be ascertained without knowing the details of their religion and can be asked with the same respect for differences and search for similarities as for other health parameters.

Using methods of respectful questioning such as the Cultural Awareness Tool (Chapter 2) may assist the practitioner in finding out about how the patient's spiritual beliefs affect their physical and mental health.

The health professional may practise the same religion as the patient, but should be aware that not everyone from the 'same' religion has the same values and practices. For example, the Roman Catholic Church is strictly against the use of artificial means of contraception, while many practising and devout Catholics will use the oral contraceptive pill or condoms. (This in fact may lead to distress amongst patients who feel that they are going against their religion but have good reasons to do so.) While many professionals will have some knowledge of the major religions, they may be sceptical and disparaging of what is felt to be outside the establishment, such as New Age, mentioned above.

Those professionals who do practise a religion will know of the benefits of ritual and adhering to a code of conduct that guides their lives. Those who do not need to be open to their patients' sources of comfort and not judge or criticise but help them to explore their religious beliefs and discover new meaning and nourishment in them.

BOX 6.8 CASE STUDY 5 (MOHAMMED'S STORY)

Mohammed came to say goodbye. He had come to Australia as a refugee full of hope and courage. Now his hopes had finally been dashed. He had not seen his wife or children since leaving his home in Iraq in the middle of the night 10 years ago. He had made the risky journey to Australia and spent three years in detention. After two more years he was still on a Temporary Protection Visa so could not sponsor them to come to Australia and could not leave the country to see them. He was afraid for their safety in Iran, as he had heard that the government was sending people back across the border. He was tired and had angina, his diabetes was out of control and now for the third time his family had been refused refugee status in their own right. He had been sure that Allah would grant him his wish. He said he had lost his faith and had decided that life could not go on. He was disappointed with Allah and felt that he was a failure as a husband and father. His faith had been the main reason he had been able to keep going all of this time.

The doctor, a Christian woman, asked him to tell her about Allah and how his faith had kept him going in the past. He talked about hope, about how every time he knelt to pray he knew that Allah was near and would keep him safe, how Allah kept his promises to those who followed his ways. At the end of the consultation both doctor and patient were crying. Mohammed thanked the doctor for showing him the way back to life. He again knew that his faith would sustain him and that Allah would keep him strong. He was not going to kill himself.

The doctor knew that her best CBT skills and most powerful medication would not have helped Mohammed. Only a spiritual discussion was going to save his life. When his wife and family finally joined him a year later, Mohammed proudly brought them to see her and they both quietly shed another tear.

Providing healthcare with a spiritual focus includes engaging with patients 'who are trying to make sense of the circumstances they find themselves in, in their search for answers to ultimate questions'.[20] To do this, health professionals cannot be detached or remote from their patients – the old-fashioned way of being objective and not getting involved with patients' feelings. But by becoming more involved in holistic and spiritual care, the professional is also at risk of emotional distress and needs to be aware of self-care and debriefing issues.

PRACTICAL POINTS
➤ Resilience is a protective factor against developing mental health problems.
➤ Therapy can help patients develop resilience.
➤ Health professionals need to explore the spiritual aspects of their patients' lives as appropriate.
➤ Spirituality is not necessarily confined to the traditional major world religions but encompasses New Age mysticism and personal beliefs.

REFERENCES
1 Nouwen H. *Reaching Out*. New York: Doubleday; 1975.
2 Luthans F. The need for and meaning of positive organizational behaviour. *J Organ Behav*. 2001; **23**: 695–706.
3 Deveson A. *Resilience*. Sydney: Allen & Unwin; 2003.
4 World Health Organization. 2007 *Mental Health: strengthening mental health promotion*. Available at: www.who.int/mediacentre/factsheets/fs220/en/ (accessed April 2008).
5 Australian Indigenous HealthInfoNet. *What is the Australian Indigenous HealthInfoNet?* 2008. Available at: www.healthinfonet.ecu.edu.au/html/html_home/home_aboutus.htm (accessed April 2008).
6 Marsella A. Culture and psychopathology. In: Kitayama S, Cohen D, editors. *Handbook of Cultural Psychology*. New York, Guilford Publications, Inc; 2007. pp. 797–818.
7 Marsella A, Yamada A. Culture and mental health: an introduction and overview of foundations, concepts, and issues. In: Cuellar I, Paniagua F, editors. *Handbook of Multicultural Mental Health*. New York, Academic Press; 2000. pp. 3–24.

8 Kaufman J, Yang B, Douglas-Palumberi H, *et al.* Brain-derived neurotrophic factor-5-HTTLPR gene interactions and environmental modifiers of depression in children. *Biol Psychiatry.* 2006; **59**: 673–80.

9 Eckersley R. Culture, spirituality, religion and health: looking at the big picture. *Med J Aust.* 2007; **186**(Suppl. 10): S54–6.

10 Young-Eisendrath P. *The Resilient Spirit.* New York: Da Capo Press; 1996.

11 D'Souza R, George K. Spirituality, religion and psychiatry: its application to clinical practice. *Australas Psychiatry.* 2006; **14**: 408–12.

12 Mishler EG. Viewpoint: critical perspectives on the biomedical model. In: Mishler EG, Amarasingham LR, Hauser ST, *et al.*, editors. *Social Contexts of Health, Illness and Patient Care.* Cambridge: Cambridge University Press; 1981.

13 Engel GL. A unified concept of health and disease. *Perspect Biol Med.* 1960; **3**: 459–85.

14 Engel GL. The clinical application of the biopsychosocial model. *Am J Psychiatry.* 1980; **137**: 535–43.

15 Maslow AH. *Towards a Psychology of Being.* 3rd ed. New York: John Wiley & Sons; 1968.

16 Williams D, Sternthal M. Spirituality, religion and health: evidence and research directions. *Med J Aust.* **186**(Suppl. 10): 10: S47–50.

17 The Royal College of Psychiatrists. *Spirituality and Mental Health.* 2006. Available at: www.rcpsych.ac.uk/mentalhealthinformation/therapies/spiritualityandmentalhealth. aspx (accessed July 2007).

18 McKnight M. *How Crystals Work. Metaphysical Guide to Choosing Crystals and Minerals for Alternative Healing.* The Crystal Ball Inc. Available at: www.wehug.com/crystal-stone-healing/alternative-crystal-healing.html (accessed July 2007).

19 Lo B, Quill T, Tulsky J. Discussing palliative care with patients. *Ann Inter Med.* 1999; **130**: 744–9.

20 Greenstreet W. Spiritual care. In: Greenstreet W, editor. *Integrating Spirituality in Health and Social Care.* Oxford: Radcliffe Medical Press; 2006. p. 52.

SECTION C

Putting cultural mental health into context

7

The people: doctors, health professionals and patients from diverse backgrounds

This chapter explores:
- Who are international medical graduates?
- Health professional migration
- Issues relating to professional language
- Health culture and health literacy
- Acculturation and culture shock
- Racism in health

In any patient–health professional interaction there are at least two people. Either or both of these may be from a different country than the one in which the consultation is taking place and/or they may be from two very different cultural backgrounds. How much does this affect the interaction? Are any problems that arise from such interactions similar to those in which there are gender or age differences? How is country of origin and/or cultural background a defining feature of what takes place?

In this chapter we consider how people are more regularly crossing borders, their motivations to do so and how this multiculturalism is affecting healthcare. There are issues to consider of social and health equity, politics and communication. The number of people involved in migration is staggering – in 2000 the United Nations estimated that 175 million people were living outside their country of origin.[1] We can expect that all of these migrants will need to seek healthcare at one time or another. For some it will be easy, for others it will be logistically and/or financially difficult. A proportion will be health professionals moving to look for work, wishing to undergo specialist training, hoping for increased remuneration or fleeing political/social upheaval.

INTERNATIONAL MEDICAL GRADUATES (IMGs)

Figures vary from different sources but approximately 23–25% of doctors in Canada, USA[2] and Australia[3] are IMGs and over 28% in the UK; while in 2004, 44% of the new registrations in the UK were from countries other than the UK or other EEA countries.[4] Many of these doctors are likely to begin their medical careers in their new country in areas of need, often in rural areas. For example, in Australia about 65% of IMGs are working in locations outside capital cities.[5] The 2007 General Practice Education and Training (GPET) figures revealed that 34% of the new general practice registrars in that year were IMGs and another 29% were Australian-trained doctors born overseas. The IMGs were typically older, with an average age of 40.[6] There are also a large number of overseas medical students in UK and Australian medical schools, often from Asia, Africa and the Indian subcontinent. It is also important to remember that 25% of the Australian, 18.4% of the Canadian and 8.3% of the UK general population have been born overseas. The countries of origin are likely to be different for doctors, students, refugees and migrants. Those born overseas are at risk of carrying a greater burden of psychosocial problems than their home-born counterparts.

For many years being in possession of a medical qualification meant that doctors and nurses were able to travel and practise around the world – sometimes even language barriers did not prevent this. However, most countries will now only accept medical degrees from other countries that have a reciprocal agreement about medical registration. Usually such agreements occur when medical training is similar in length and quality. If a doctor wishes to practise in a country where there is no agreement about his or her qualification, the doctor must undergo some form of competency testing – often both a written and clinical examination.

While doctors from developed resource-rich countries sometimes wish to work for a while in a developing country to gain new skills and/or for altruistic reasons, there is a huge drain of qualified doctors in the opposite direction, from developing countries to the resource rich. The attrition rate of trained mental health workers in developing countries is a great problem because of issues such as geographic and professional isolation.[7] Doctors in the developed world earn more than their poorer cousins and it is easy to see the attraction of moving from a war-torn or famine-struck country to what is imagined as a land of plenty. It is not only the remuneration that is attractive, but also less bureaucracy and more equality of opportunity in medical careers. In the developed countries there is usually no shortage of access to investigations or drugs and doctors are able to offer their patients more choice and enable them to live longer. Moreover, the doctors' families are able to live in better conditions, with schooling and healthcare provided (though in some cases they may have to pay for these). With increased income, doctors are also able to send money 'back home' to their extended families. In 2000 about 30% of NHS staff were such 'medical migrants'.[8]

There is a shortage of doctors in the developed world and there is a workforce crisis in rural and remote areas of richer nations. These countries encourage doctors to move and work within their medical workforce and, while there is some support, there are often cultural and communication barriers between doctor and patient. The Association of Medical Faculties of Canada has addressed the difficulties of integrating IMGs into their workforce by developing a series of online modules so that teachers and supervisors can be better prepared for their work with IMGs. They acknowledge that IMGs are a valuable and diverse group with learning needs that are likely to differ from other Canadians.[2]

The ethics of poor nations educating doctors only to lose them to their richer neighbours are often ignored. This one-way flow does little to ease global health inequalities. As one Indian-born and trained psychiatrist now working in the UK writes: 'Consider, for example, a country that must import expatriate doctors using scarce foreign exchange. Most doctors in developing countries have been trained in public funded medical schools. The cost of training is borne by the poor country and the rich country reaps the benefits. In effect, the people of poor countries are paying for the healthcare of those who live in one of the richest.'[9]

Of course, doctors also come to richer nations for postgraduate training and in the UK were able to do so until recently without needing work permits under the Highly Skilled Migrant Programme. Such doctors were promised permanent residency status after four years, but the British Government tried to renege on this promise, meaning that these non-EU doctors would be the last in line for training-post positions. This change would have prevented doctors from outside the EU entering British training posts if there were suitable candidates for such posts from the UK and EU.[10] This development of course outraged overseas doctors, as the UK has for many years relied on them for bolstering the National Health Service in times of doctor shortages. The recent increase in medical student numbers in the UK is predicted to overcome these shortages and therefore overseas-trained doctors were thought to be no longer necessary. However, the Court of Appeal in November 2007 has ruled that such discrimination is unlawful and that all appropriately qualified doctors should be able to compete for training posts.[11] There are similar issues in other developed countries – each with its own political overtones. Thus the cultural background of doctors will continue to be diverse, and cultural awareness continues to be of prime importance within the health service.

One example of the issues caused by such medical migration is that of Timor Leste and Cuba. Cuba is one of the greatest exporters of medical doctors in the world. Currently 36 578 Cuban doctors work in 73 nations.[12] In Timor Leste, the Cuban Medical Brigade has provided much-needed healthcare throughout the country. However, the Cubans and people from Timor Leste have no language in common and there are also concerns about cultural sensitivity and the quality of care in terms of local needs.[13]

THE ETHNIC MIX OF DOCTORS

Figures relating to the ethnic profile of doctors in the UK make interesting reading. In 2003 in England 63% were white, 23% Asian, 4% black, 1% of mixed race and 7% from other ethnic groups (2% unrecorded) – this is in comparison to the overall population in which 92% of people are white.[14] The difference is partly related to the immigration into the UK of overseas-trained doctors with different national, cultural and religious backgrounds. However, the medical profession is a highly regarded career choice amongst British-born students of Asian descent. These UK-trained doctors will have different attitudes and values to overseas doctors as a result of their medical programme, but will also have their own cultural heritage as a factor in patient–doctor interactions.

The importance of this mix is that often patient and doctor will have differing values, often differing first languages and differing health beliefs. However, the danger is in assuming these differences on the basis of appearance. As highlighted many times in this book, the fundamental basis of the interaction must be patient-centred with exploration of views and beliefs. But patients must also put aside prejudices of their own and learn about their doctor's professional behaviour through communication. There may be insurmountable obstacles relating to understanding, particularly in consultations where mental health is a focus. However, such difficulties are not always ethnically propagated. Culture is a factor – maybe as simple as the gap in age between an elderly doctor who abhors the thought of recreational drugs and a 20-something party animal who sees no problems with the odd ecstasy tablet or puff of cannabis.

Aneez Esmail, professor of general practice at the University of Manchester, writes eloquently of the history of Asian doctors in the NHS, recounting that when overseas-trained doctors became commonplace in the UK, there were many complaints about communication problems. However, objective testing showed this to be only an issue for a minority of doctors and that these problems disappeared within three years. Professor Esmail feels that blaming language and the subsequent belief that overseas doctors practise a poor standard of care is a form of racism. Such racism leads to all overseas doctors eventually becoming stigmatised. Esmail writes: 'The irony of course is that most GPs know that communication is not just about language and intonation and not knowing the right words. It is as much an issue about class and culture and recognizing that perhaps the greatest barrier of communication is the culture of biomedicine rather than the culture of your spoken language' (p. 831).[15]

PROFESSIONAL LANGUAGE

Eliciting a history from a patient, exploring ideas, concerns, expectations and health beliefs, discussing a diagnosis, formulating a management plan and sharing decisions with patients are professional interactions between the healthcare provider and the patient. The health professional should ensure that such communication is intelligible and use minimal professional jargon in professional conversations with people seeking help or advice.

BOX 7.1 HEALTH PROFESSIONAL DISCOURSE[17]

- Personal experience discourse is talk concerned with the individual's experiences and feelings. It usually takes the form of a narrative (anecdotes, reminiscences, etc) and deals with the 'here and now experience of the concrete particulars of a case in hand' and 'the accumulated experience of a similar case over time'.[16]
- Professional discourse is the talk of doctors in practice, exemplified in doctor–patient interviews, in case rounds in hospitals and in a range of doctor–doctor discussions and meetings. It is the discourse of shared ways of knowing and seeing that characterise the community of medical practitioners.
- Institutional discourse is not the actual talk that doctors use in their consultations (that is, professional discourse); rather it is the ways in which doctors account for this talk. In other words, the everyday competencies and practices of the doctor have to be presented in institutional terms

through language that reifies and abstracts these practices, e.g. clinical practice meetings. The dominance of institutional discourse over other forms of discourse is maintained through typical institutional encounters such as selection examinations, departmental meetings and quality assessments that hold institutions together both politically and organisationally.

Three types of discourse have been identified as occurring in the daily lives of health professionals (Box 7.1).[17] Interactions between health professionals, *professional discourse*, often take the form of shorthand, with the liberal use of abbreviations and acronyms. Sometimes such professional conversations are misunderstood because of the use of profession- or discipline-specific jargon. This is important when considering referrals, particularly of patients with mental health problems to other agencies, counsellors, psychologists, psychiatrists, community psychiatric nurses etc, if such discourse is ambiguous or misconstrued. Even our definitions of the people we interact with differ from profession to profession. Medically we consult with patients, but in some circumstances they may be clients, service users, even consumers. If we ask the 'patient' what she wants to be called, she may well reply 'Mrs. Smith' or 'Patricia'.

Doctors with English as a second/other language (ESOL) have been shown to be disadvantaged particularly in relation to institutional language and this may affect their performance in oral assessments.[17] This difficulty may translate into problems when overseas-trained professionals are mentored or supported while providing counselling to patients. Describing a patient's feelings and experiences by translating them into professional or institutional language may be difficult for an ESOL person, who may have elicited an excellent history, but who may then have trouble putting the patient's language into that expected by colleagues.

However, there is a converse side to this. Often students and inexperienced staff slip into professional discourse when talking to patients. They elicit histories in the standard form using institutional discourse then to present the case: 'a 72-year-old retired farmer presented to the Emergency Department with worsening depression and suicidal intent'. Clinical educators do well to ask the students to describe the patient's symptoms in his or her own words.

INTERNATIONAL MEDICAL GRADUATES – ISSUES AROUND ORIENTATION

The orientation period for IMGs is often short and concentrates on the immediate job that the IMG is about to start. There may be an introduction to the hospital system, how to order investigations and prescribing, there may even be some discussion about the working of the National Health Service (or the health service of the country to which the doctor has migrated) and the fact that healthcare is free at the point of delivery (which may be very different from the situation in the doctor's own country) but there is likely to be little exploration of the patient's journey within the NHS and the diversity of beliefs within the same country. Doctors learn by experience. Doctors who trained in the country in which they practise also learn from every patient with whom they interact. However, many junior doctors say they feel unprepared for their first day on the wards – imagine then the perplexity of a newly arrived doctor who has to cope not only with a new health delivery system, but also with a population of comparative strangers.

In the UK, as a result of the opting out by GPs of after-hours calls, many non-British-trained doctors are working at night and at weekends. These unsocial hours are when patients are often at their most vulnerable and the number of health professionals that a doctor may call on for support is limited.

BOX 7.2 CASE STUDY 1 (MEDICAL MIGRATION)

Dr Krishnan trained and qualified as a medical doctor in Madras (Chennai). In India he practised as a general surgeon following specialist training. He worked a 14-hour day in a public hospital and rarely had time to see his wife and two small children. His income, while higher than the majority of his patients, was low. He answered an advertisement for doctors in Australia. Due to the registration regulations he is not able to be recognised as a surgeon but is able to work in a rural town in outback Queensland as a general practitioner with procedural skills. He is on-call most of the time but the day-to-day workload is not excessive. As his medical training was mostly in English, he has good communication skills but cannot always understand his Australian patients and they cannot always understand him. This is frustrating, particularly as some patients question his diagnoses and management, a situation almost unheard of in his previous practice. After a month settling in, his family came to join him in this land of opportunity. His wife is slow to acclimatise; she cannot get used to the 'bigness' of the land and the lack of people. She has become depressed, which impacts on Dr Krishnan's own well-being.

Dr Krishnan's wife may not have the opportunity or desire to see a doctor in the same town. Dr Krishnan meanwhile has to cope with the stresses that his patients bring to him. Any stress that he has because of his own or his wife's situation is likely to interfere with his ability to interact with his patients, especially with the cultural barriers that are already in place.

This case highlights some of the problems associated with migration. Registration bodies cannot simply look at a doctor's qualifications and language skills but need to consider his/her family situation – there needs to be an holistic assessment of the doctor's suitability for practice just as health professionals should be making holistic assessments of their patients' well-being.

INTERACTIONS BETWEEN MENTALLY UNWELL PATIENTS AND HEALTH PROFESSIONALS IN FAMILIAR AND 'FOREIGN' HEALTHCARE SYSTEMS

Negotiating one's way through a country's healthcare system is difficult. This is the case for both migrant health professionals and patients. Doctors need to understand how to prescribe and how much drugs will cost patients. They need to be aware of medical certification for taking time off work and how to refer suicidal or aggressive patients. When a doctor is unclear about the system, he or she becomes more anxious when interacting with patients, especially if patients appear to be asking for certain drugs about which doctors have reservations. It is easy to become suspicious about a patient who is asking for benzodiazepines, sleeping tablets or strong painkillers. Such suspicion directed to a patient with mental health problems may further undermine the patient's fragile state. For registered patients in the UK there should be good clinical records to help when patients move between doctors. Patient records after hours or in some countries are often incomplete. There is the potential for misunderstanding and inappropriate prescribing (either giving or refusing to give medication).

Doctors from certain developing countries who undertake assessment of competence in order to be able to practise in Australia, for example, often have problems in reaching the required standard for interactions with patients with mental health problems. This raises interesting questions about medical training and illness prevalence in the doctors' countries of origin.

For patients there are many factors that reduce their access to healthcare (Box 7.3). General practices and health centres should ensure that their services, appointment systems and reception staff are accessible to the community they serve. Information about services should be available in appropriate languages. People from culturally diverse backgrounds should be encouraged to join patient participation groups and their communities should be invited to have a say in timing and availability of health services.

BOX 7.3 FACTORS THAT REDUCE ACCESS TO HEALTHCARE

- Language proficiency.
- Family responsibilities.
- Types of appointment systems.
- Timing of appointments.
- Social isolation.
- Access to transport.
- Cost (real or perceived).
- Cultural restrictions regarding movement of women in public spaces.
- Cultural restrictions on education and employment for women.
- Cultural imperatives for women to see female health workers.

HEALTH CULTURE AND HEALTH LITERACY

Every society has a particular 'culture' related to health, as it has to relationships, transition to adulthood, birth, death, family hierarchy and so on. This cultural domain will often have built up over many generations and like the other aspects of society will change over time as other parameters change. The influences on the culture of health may come from within, such as changing disease patterns and birthing rituals, or from outside, such as the influence of Western biological paradigms and medication. The language and advice from interactions with health professionals is fed back over time into the patient's own cultural system, so that within any community there is a gradient from the more traditional views of health and illness to the more scientific ideas of the host country[18] (and vice versa if migration is from a Western culture). 'Symptoms and signs' that have previously been part of a spiritual or social framework may be taken up by health or may move from health into another framework. This is particularly evident for mental health issues. Schizophrenia, for example, is viewed as a spiritual problem in many cultures and in the 1970s in Western society was seen as a family issue. Freud saw hysteria as the outcome of sexual difficulties, and personality disorders are commonly viewed as the outcome of family or social dysfunction. Societies through the ages have labelled those who are socially 'unacceptable' as having a mental illness and have used this as a means of social control.

The treatment of psychological and psychiatric illness will follow from the cultural view of its aetiology. For example, if it is seen as a spiritual issue, it may need a priest; if a family difficulty, a family counsellor; if a sexual problem, a sex therapist; if stemming from the community, an elder may be needed to help solve the problem; if a social misfit, the criminal justice system might be involved. The 'medicalisation' of mental health will engender strong reactions in many who believe that psychological, family and societal issues need to be addressed and that the biomedical model is inappropriate.

The 'health culture' of many societies is now embracing a combination of traditional, spiritual, psychosocial and biomedical models to both explain and treat mental illness. This does not necessarily mean that the practitioners of the various models embrace each other, but that the culture itself has a tacit acceptance that mental health is a complex issue involving many different facets of life. Antipathy between various types of practitioners in any society means that patients will sometimes be loath to admit they are seeking help from a variety of different sources. Unless the treatment is dangerous, as in some cases of exorcism for mental health problems where patients have died, a practitioner should acknowledge the strong cultural pull to use an explanatory model outside health.

As with other aspects of culture, 'health culture' is mostly unconscious, both in the practitioner and in the patient. 'Ethnocentrism' is the normal tendency of an individual to view his or herself, others and the world from the viewpoint of his or her own culture or subculture. This is mostly unconscious and a health professional's initial assessment of a patient, illness or situation will always be from his or her own upbringing or culture. More than in any other area of medicine the 'ethnocentrism' of the mental health practitioner needs to be made conscious so that the cultural beliefs and expectations of the patient can be properly addressed. Patience, acceptance, a strong therapeutic alliance and flexibility of treatment options are of the utmost importance so the cultural stance of the patient can be objectively explored. To treat what a patient sees as a spiritual problem with medication or to treat with family therapy what the patient sees as a physical issue will ensure non-compliance and confusion. If possible, a multifactorial explanation of aetiology and a balance and inclusiveness of all treatments should be negotiated.

In Western society, alternative therapies have become more and more socially acceptable, with a high proportion of patients using alternative therapy instead of, or alongside, their usual medical treatment. Some of these therapies, for example glucosamine for arthritis, have been taken up by allopathic (conventional) medicine because the appropriate level of 'evidence' through research has proven their benefits.

'Health literacy' is a term mostly used to describe a patient's understanding of their health. Western doctors usually refer to this as an understanding of anatomy, physiology and the pathological basis of disease. This is important if investigations or treatment such as medication or surgery are recommended. Health promotion, epidemiology and evidence-based medicine are concepts that guide good medical practice throughout the world. Everyone is entitled to have access to such care, and organisations such as the World Health Organization are committed to a high level of evidence-based medicine being universally available. It needs to be remembered that the evidence in one culture or ethnic group cannot necessarily be extrapolated to another. Such a definition of health literacy does not take into account the different cultural understanding and expectations of health. This other type of health literacy involves at least an acknowledgement that, as with any type of literacy, it does not just involve the 'scientific' knowledge of a concept but also the more elusive overlying cultural narrative. This then becomes a learning process for all concerned – for the health professional to become more literate in the patient's understanding of health and for the patient to become more literate in that of the health professional.

It is understandable that those who are working across cultures struggle to fully grasp how the 'health culture' of the patient is influencing their current illness. In order to develop a strong therapeutic alliance there will need to be a respect for the differences from both sides; a commitment to learning as much about each other's 'health culture' as is necessary for the current therapeutic encounter; an agreement on the desired outcomes; and a flexibility of options that may involve both evidence-based and traditional aspects. Such a task is complex and time-consuming but without it a consultation may be unintelligible to one of the parties and be of no use. For those who are practising outside their original culture, it may mean being constantly alert to the subtle health messages given by patients, but also by the society via multimedia such as television and advertisements.

Seemingly insurmountable difficulties will occur when different cultural understandings seem to be mutually exclusive. Nowhere is this more evident than with mental health issues. For instance, the growing body of evidence about the changes in brain anatomy, physiology and biochemistry seen in different mental illnesses brings with it evidence of the comparative efficacy of medication and psychotherapy. A practitioner armed with the latest literature may meet what feels like stubborn opposition from a patient who comes from a culture that views mental illness as a spiritual problem, who has a fatalistic view of life or who believes that mental processes and personalities are inherently immutable. This is likely to be more evident when trying to convey the changes that are seen in the brain with psychotherapy. Attempting to assist such a patient using cognitive behavioural therapy (CBT) for instance, especially if discussing challenging core beliefs, is likely to meet misunderstanding or even open resistance.

Patients and therapists alike may struggle to simultaneously hold opposing cultural views of aetiology or treatment of a mental health disorder. The internal conflict generated by divergent cultural views may even be part of the original problem that has brought a patient to see a health practitioner. On the other hand, the evolution of a multicultural view of life and psychological well-being may assist with the patient's integration. For practitioners this might cause difficulties learning new skills in psychotherapy because of conscious or unconscious resistance to the new concepts.

How culture influences health

While a person's health beliefs are strongly shaped by their culture and upbringing, there are other influences under the heading of 'culture' that may not be so obvious. MacLachlan has developed a taxonomy of how culture interplays with health (Box 7.4).[19] An understanding of history is important to realise the impact of colonialism and its effects on certain groups. The aftermath of empire building is still evident in patterns of migration and cultural exchange, while the subtleties of attitudes to difference may not be so apparent despite their effects on help-seeking and health delivery. Cultural alternativism acknowledges the trend of many in the developed world seeking help from those who would in their own cultures have been known as traditional healers. Thus we incorporate yoga, crystal therapy and aryuvedic practice into the 'mainstream', though often separating such modalities from their underlying philosophy. Cultural evolution is similar to acculturation and acknowledges that culture changes over time.

BOX 7.4 THE INTERPLAY OF CULTURE AND HEALTH[19]

- Cultural colonialism – the dominant group compares itself to those who are 'different'.
- Cultural sensitivity – being sensitive to the needs of the people with whom we interact.
- Cultural migration – management of the health of people who move to new locations – protection of their health and that of the 'host' population.
- Cultural alternativism – awareness of less conventional approaches to healthcare, including complementary therapies.
- Cultural empowerment – cultural awakening as a type of therapy.

- Cultural globalisation – Western colonialism rebranded in financial terms.
- Cultural evolution – the effects of culture change on health within a society.

DIFFERENCE BETWEEN REFUGEES AND MIGRANTS

The 1951 United Nations Refugee Convention defines a refugee as 'A person who is outside his or her country of nationality or habitual residence; has a well-founded fear of persecution because of his or her race, religion, nationality, membership of a particular social group or political opinion; and is unable or unwilling to avail himself or herself of the protection of that country, or to return there, for fear of persecution.'[20]

There are approximately 20 million refugees in the world, fleeing their own countries because of war, ethnic cleansing or starvation. There are another 20 million internally displaced people not counted as refugees.[21] Refugees leave their country against their will. They are likely to suffer multiple losses, trauma, chaos, fear, danger, torture, illness and starvation. During their flight they will have limited access to healthcare, food or clean water and are without home, family, country, privacy or community. On making it to 'safety', they may spend long periods of time in refugee camps, in detention or as illegal immigrants, where they remain very vulnerable and their future continues to be uncertain.

There is an increase in mental health problems in refugees due to pre-flight, flight, refugee camp and resettlement factors. Up to 60% will have depression, post-traumatic stress disorder (PTSD) or anxiety disorders.[21] Children who have grown up in war-torn countries and refugee camps and especially those who have been in detention also have increases in developmental delay, behaviour problems and personality disorders such as oppositional defiant personality disorder.[22] It will be difficult to recover from PTSD if there continues to be trauma from settlement issues, intergenerational problems, domestic violence, discrimination in the new country, poverty, racism or confusion. Recovery is complex and can only really take place within the context of relationships.[23] For some, the complications of settling become overwhelming and they yearn for their country of origin and their families. Some people may return home, even though it's unsafe, because they miss their previous employment, family, religion or culture.

Migrants, on the other hand, make a conscious decision to leave their countries, usually for economic, educational or employment reasons. They will have time to plan and will be able to bring possessions and family with them and may begin making connections in the new country. Some have argued that only the best and strongest choose to migrate. However, if the pressures of migration and settling into the new culture exceed the resources available for coping, psychological problems may occur.[24] Older migrants may struggle with language, loneliness, dislocation, intergenerational differences and the prospect of never being able to visit their homeland again.[25]

Both refugees and migrants seek hope and opportunity, but often find rejection and despair that may lead to anger, paranoia and depression.[24] They may suffer from culture shock in the first few months after arrival. This is a syndrome of symptoms that include paranoia, anxiety, somatic complaints and an idealisation of the home culture.[24] After the initial 'honeymoon' phase is over, many may be faced with a reality that does not live up to their expectations. This will include unemployment, poverty, discrimination, racism, inadequate housing, lack of health services and non-recognition of occupational qualifications.[26] Migration involves many changes and challenges that a person must meet if they are to cope in the new environment. The circumstances in the new country are the most powerful stressors likely to increase the risk of mental illness.[26]

ACCULTURATION AND CULTURE SHOCK

(*See also* Chapter 11.)

Acculturation is the process of learning to live within another culture and the exchange of cultural features between peoples. This means therefore that not only migrants, but also indigenous peoples, grapple with acculturation following colonisation or land seizure. Customs of the dominant culture are also susceptible to change. (A very simple example of this is the fact that anglicised 'Indian food' in the UK has become the most popular takeaway, supplanting the British fish and chips.[27]) Acculturation is not a recently described phenomenon; in fact the word can be traced back to Plato (348 BC), who argued that the process should be minimised but not to the extent of cultural isolation.[28] The experience may be predominantly positive, with forging of new intercultural relationships and development of new skills; or negative, ranging from temporary culture shock to continuing identity crisis. The time taken to become acculturated will depend on the person's age, education level and personality. It will also be more difficult if they have come from a collectivist culture to a very different individualistic culture or vice versa.

Though the Oxford dictionary's definition of acculturation is: 'assimilate to a different culture, typically the dominant one' and assimilate is 'absorb and integrate (people, ideas or culture)',[29] acculturation should not be viewed synonymously with assimilation, the latter word having negative connotations of people having to shed their cultural heritage and become absorbed into the culture of their host country.[30] Assimilation is probably not completely possible, as subtle cultural traces are always likely to stay. More realistic and perhaps healthier is the development of a 'third culture personality' that retains basic ethnic identity and culture while at the same time coming to respect and understand the values of the new country.[31,32] This concept of a 'third culture' should help health professionals balance the patient's cultural past with their difficulties in the present and the potential richness of their future.

The literature relating to acculturation, migration and related topics is immense and spans the disciplines of anthropology, social science, psychology and economics, amongst others. There are three theories that attempt to explain the impact of migration on health and well-being (Box 7.5).

BOX 7.5 IMPACT OF MIGRATION ON HEALTH[33]

- The 'migration-morbidity' hypothesis – migrants would be expected to have worse mental health than their host society due to pre- and post-migration stressors.
- The 'health migrant' effect – people in good health are more likely to meet eligibility criteria and to be willing and economically able to migrate. Immigrant children and young people may have the ability to switch between identities, languages and cultural norms, giving them greater flexibility.
- The 'transition effect' – the health advantage that some migrant groups show disappears over time, e.g. cardiovascular risk, cancer and psychological outcomes.

There are differences of opinion as to how people from different cultures may best live together and relate to the dominant culture. Four strategies have been described but these are given different names and emphases depending on whether they are defined by the immigrant or the receiving community (Box 7.6).[34] Integration, the maintenance of one's own culture while interacting with the dominant group, has been shown to be linked to better mental health outcomes.[23] However, of course, choice of strategy is not always possible and depends on the willingness of both parties and opportunities for interactions at school, at work and in social situations. The receiving community needs to demonstrate low levels of prejudice and racism and offer equal opportunities and social equity.

BOX 7.6 FOUR STRATEGIES FOR ACCULTURATION

Migrant group	Receiving community
Integration	Multiculturalism
Assimilation	Melting pot
Separation	Segregation
Marginalisation	Exclusion

Everyone who moves country will experience some degree of culture shock, including both patients and professionals. The extent of this will depend upon a number of factors (Box 7.7).

BOX 7.7 FACTORS AFFECTING CULTURE SHOCK

- Migration being voluntary or forced.
- Language – the same or different, expertise in new language.
- Climate and physical demands of this.
- Financial security.
- Housing.
- Support networks – family and friends in new country.
- Work – unemployment or looking for work is more stressful than moving to a new job.
- Dress and customs.
- Food and hygiene practices.
- Knowledge and availability of healthcare.
- Knowledge and availability of education.
- Recognition of qualifications from home country.

Culture shock and subsequent mental health problems are more likely in groups who are forced to move home or change lifestyles, e.g. refugees or first nations, than in groups who choose to migrate, e.g. economic migrants. However, people who choose to relocate may have unrealistic visions of their new home and their expectations may be shattered, leading to subsequent ill health. Settling in a new country usually moves through a process of a honeymoon phase, the phase of culture shock, a phase where integration into the new community is taking place and finally a phase of acceptance occurs.

Helping the acculturation process

Three major conceptual frameworks, derived from social and health psychology, have been described that help professionals understand the process of acculturation and its potential problems and challenges (Box 7.8).[23] When the process is difficult, people may seek help from health professionals. But the problems and challenges apply equally to health professionals working within new systems and cultures themselves.

BOX 7.8 HELPING ACCULTURATION

- **Affective components** – stress and coping framework: acculturation is a series of stress-provoking life events and changes requiring adaptation and coping responses
  — *Strategies to help* – problem-focussed strategies and social support.
- **Behavioural elements** – culture learning approach
  — *Strategies to help* – learning specific skills to cope with everyday life, e.g. learning the language to avoid isolation.
- **Cognitive variables** – establishing social identity
  — *Strategies to help* – having two cultural identities causes conflict, e.g. home and social life.

The stress and coping framework arises from the knowledge that major life changes such as divorce or bereavement may cause mental ill health and that adjustment is required. Moving house is also a major life stress and moving across cultures is even more so. Focussing on problems such as planning for the change and arranging social support, rather than withdrawal into one's own territory and disengaging from the new culture, is helpful.

Learning about the new culture and the necessary skills to function within it are important. Things that we take for granted become more difficult in a new society where the rules may be different, and institutional requirements vary. Language is an important skill as is appropriate transcultural training, depending on profession.

Living in a new culture means having to learn to deal with two identities, especially if the person is working or being educated within the new country. This is an issue also for second- and third-generation children who may feel they have to choose between their family culture and the culture in which they are immersed outside the home.

BOX 7.9 CASE STUDY 2 (MEDICAL MIGRATION)

Dr Hosseini is a GP registrar in his first practice post. He qualified in Iran and came to the UK as a political refugee. He passed the appropriate assessments and was eventually accepted onto a general practice vocational training scheme. Today the registrars are discussing palliative care at their half-day release educational session and are working through scenarios with the help of simulated patients. Dr Hosseini is consulting with Mary Foster, a 43-year-old single mother who has metastatic ovarian cancer. She has moved from her previous home to live with her sister, as she can no longer cope by herself while trying to look after her 10-year-old son. She wants to talk about the available care in her new location and to renew her prescription for analgesia. Dr Hosseini is considerate and listens to Mary's anxieties in relation to dying and leaving her son on his own. Dr Hosseini agrees to refer her to the local palliative care team. He also suggests that she might want to talk to her priest in order to prepare herself for death. Mary says that she is not religious and has no need for spiritual care. Dr Hosseini insists that a priest would be helpful for her and that she should consider her religious beliefs before she dies. Mary is distressed by this insistence. In the debrief for the session the registrar group discuss the role of religion in palliative care and agree that it is important for a GP to explore a patient's beliefs about dying and a possible afterlife. Dr Hosseini is upset because he feels that any person without religion will struggle towards the end of life and he felt he was doing the best for his patient. He is a devout Muslim and is aware that not all British people go to church, but had thought that almost all should be Christian by upbringing.

RACISM AND ITS EFFECTS ON INTERACTIONS

The Macpherson report into the murder of London teenager Stephen Lawrence defines institutional racism as:

> The collective failure of an organisation to provide an appropriate and professional service to people because of their colour, culture or ethnic origin. It can be seen or detected in processes, attitudes and behaviour which amount to discrimination through unwitting prejudice, ignorance, thoughtlessness and racist stereotyping which disadvantages minority ethnic people.[35]

Prejudice derives from many different sources. American psychologists suggest that it arises from four interlinked conditions (Table 7.1).[36] One study from an educational setting showed that the strongest unique predictor of a person's attitude to people from different cultural backgrounds is whether there is difficulty in communication. Such difficulty may arise from accented speech, inability to speak each other's language or differences in non-verbal communication. Lack of communication then causes discomfort, impatience and frustration, leading to prejudice.[37]

TABLE 7.1 Sources of prejudice (adapted from Stephan and Stephan[29])

Condition/source	Effect in a consultation
Negative stereotypes (cognitive beliefs)	Thinking of patients from different cultural backgrounds as lazy, arrogant, prone to psychosomatic complaints
Intergroup anxiety	Suspicious and hostile to outsiders; anxious and frustrated by an inability to understand each other and therefore help as a doctor
Realistic threats (economic and physical)	Believing that certain patients overuse health service resources to which they have not contributed; a burden on the health service
Symbolic/cultural threats	Patients undermine one's own culture and beliefs

PRACTICAL TIPS

➤ The transcultural interaction between patient and professional must be patient-centred, with exploration of views and beliefs.
➤ Both patients and professionals must put aside prejudices and learn about each other.
➤ Health professionals should ensure that communication is intelligible and use minimal professional jargon with people seeking help or advice.
➤ The cultural background of patients and doctors will continue to be diverse, and cultural awareness will continue to be of prime importance within the health service.
➤ Health professionals migrating to a new country need a period of orientation.
➤ For both patient and professions, negotiating a way through a country's healthcare system is difficult and needs patience and understanding on both sides.
➤ The 'health culture' of many societies is now embracing a combination of traditional, spiritual, psychosocial and biomedical models to both explain and treat mental illness.
➤ Everyone who moves country will experience some degree of culture shock, including both patients and professionals.

REFERENCES

1 United Nations. *World Immigration Report*. New York: UN; 2000.

2 Association of Faculties of Medicine of Canada. *A Faculty Development Program for Teachers of International Medical Graduates*. Available at: www.afmc.ca/img/default_ en.htm (accessed April 2008).

3 Hawthorne L, Hawthorne G, Crotty B. *Final Report: The Registration and Training Status of Overseas Trained Doctors in Australia*. Melbourne: The University of Melbourne; 2007.

4 General Medical Council. *Annual Review 2004/2005*. Available at: www.gmc-uk.org/ publications/annual_reports/annual_review_2004_5.pdf (accessed April 2008).

5 Pilotto L, Duncan G, Anderson-Wurf J. Issues for clinicians training international medical graduates: a systemic review. *Med J Aust*. 2007; **187**: 225–8.

6 Hingston C. GP career draws large local intake. *Aust Doct*. 9 March 2007: 2.

7 Cohen A. Nations for Mental Health. *The Effectiveness of Mental Health Services in Primary Care: the view from the developing world*. 2002. Available at: www.who.int/ mental_health/media/en/50.pdf (accessed January 2008).

8 Welsh C. Training overseas doctors in the United Kingdom. *BMJ*. 2000; **321**: 253–4.

9 Patel V. Recruiting doctors from poorer countries: the great brain robbery? *BMJ*. 2003; **327**: 926–8.

10 Dyer C. High court rejects overseas doctors' challenge of UK work restrictions. *BMJ*. 2007; **334**: 333.

11 BBC News. Overseas doctors win NHS ruling. 9 November 2007. Available at: www. news.bbc.co.uk/1/hi/health/7087846.stm (accessed November 2007).

12 Prensa Latina – Latin American News Agency. Cuban physicians to aid 81 nations. 29 March 2008. Available at: www.plenglish.com/article.asp?ID=%7B771AA7E5-B9F3-4129-AFF7-208C0DC1D65D%7D)&language=EN (accessed April 2008).

13 Zwi A, Marins J, Grove N, *et al*. *Timor-Leste: health sector resilience and performance in a time of instability. Timor-Leste Health Sector Resilience Study*. 2007. Sydney: University of New South Wales; 2007.

14 Bowler I. Ethnic profile of doctors in the United Kingdom. *BMJ*. 2004; **329**: 583–4.

15 Esmail A. Asian doctors in the NHS: service and betrayal. *BJGP*. 2007; **57**: 827–34.

16 Atkinson P. *Medical Talk and Medical Work*. London: Sage; 1995.

17 Roberts C, Sarangi S, Southgate L, *et al*. Oral examinations – equal opportunities, ethnicity, and fairness in the MRCGP. *BMJ*. 2000; **320**: 370–5.

18 Angel R, Thoits P. The impact of culture on the cognitive structure of illness. *Cult Med Psychiatry*. 1987; **11**: 465–94.

19 MacLachlan M. Culture, empowerment and health. In: Murray M, editor. *Critical Health Psychology*. Basingstoke: Palgrave Macmillan; 2004. pp. 101–17.

20 The UN Refugee Agency. *The 1951 Refugee Convention: questions and answers*. Available at: www.unhcr.org/basics/BASICS/3c0f495f4.pdf (accessed May 2008).

21 Kinzie J. Immigrants and refugees: the psychiatric perspective. *Transcult Psychiatry*. 2006; **43**: 577–91.

22 Silove D, Austin P, Steel Z. No refuge from terror: the impact of detention on the mental health of trauma-affected refugees seeking asylum in Australia. *Transcult Psychiatry*. 2007; **44**: 359–93.

23 Herman J. *Trauma and Recovery*. New York: BasicBooks; 1992.

24 Marsella A. Culture and psychopathology. In: Kitayama S, Cohen D, editors. *Handbook of Cultural Psychology*. New York: Guilford Publications, Inc; 2007. pp. 797–818.

25 Klimidis S, Stuart G, Minas H, *et al.* Immigrant status and gender effects on psychopathology and self-concept in adolescents: a test of the migration–morbidity hypothesis. *Compr Psychiatry*. 1994; **35**: 393–404.

26 Minas H, Silove D. Transcultural and refugee psychiatry. In: Bloch S, Singh B, editors. *Foundations of Clinical Psychiatry*. Melbourne, Australia: Melbourne University Press; 2001. pp. 475–90.

27 BBC News. India gets a taste of UK tikka. 3 November 1999. Available at: www.news.bbc.co.uk/1/hi/uk/503680.stm (accessed December 2007).

28 Rudmin FW. Catalogue of acculturation constructs: descriptions of 126 taxonomies, 1918–2003. In: Lonner WJ, Dinnel DL, Hayes SA, *et al.*, editors. *Online Readings in Psychology*. Available at: www.ac.wwu.edu/~culture/rudmin.htm (accessed February 2008).

29 Soanes C, Stevenson A, editors. *Oxford Dictionary of English*. 2nd ed. Oxford: Oxford University Press; 2003.

30 Ward CA. The ABCs of acculturation. In: Pedersen PB, Draguns JG, Lonner WJ, *et al.*, editors. *Counseling Across Cultures*. 6th ed. Los Angeles: Sage; 2008. pp. 291–306.

31 Benson J. *Third Culture Personalities and the Integration of Refugees into the Community: some reflections from general practice*. 2003. Available at: www.mmha.org.au/mmha-products/synergy/2003_No2/ThirdCulturePersonalities/ (accessed April 2008).

32 Gonsalves C. Psychological stages of the refugee process: a model for therapeutic interventions. *Prof Psych Res Pr*. 1992; **23**: 382–9.

33 Australian Government. *Cultural Competency in Health: a guide for policy, partnerships and participation*. Canberra: NHMRC publications; 2005.

34 Berry JW. A psychology of immigration. *J Soc Issues*. 2001; **57**: 615–31.

35 Macpherson W. *The Stephen Lawrence Inquiry Report*. London: The Stationery Office; 1999.

36 Stephan WG, Stephan CW. Predicting prejudice. *Int J Intercult Relat*. 1996; **20**: 409–26.

37 Spencer-Rodgers J, McGovern T. Attitudes toward the culturally different: the role of intercultural communication barriers, affective responses, consensual stereotypes and perceived threat. *Int J Intercult Relat*. 2002; **26**: 609–31.

8

Consultations across cultures

This chapter explores:
- Transcultural counselling
- Terminology
- Interpreters and advocates
- Initial consultations
- Patient–professional interactions
- Setting boundaries
- Physical and mental health questionnaires
- Patient partnership
- Reflecting on consultations
- Patterns of cultural differences
- The self: individualism and collectivism
- Confidentiality

Consultations across cultures occur when the patient and the health professional are from different cultural backgrounds. When counselling is part of the management strategy, this process may be referred to as 'cross' or 'inter' cultural counselling, though the prefix 'trans' may be preferred, as it emphasises 'the *active* and *reciprocal* process that is involved'.[1] The health professional, counsellor or therapist needs to acknowledge cultural differences and work with and through these. For transcultural consultations to be effective the health professional needs to integrate the interacting multiple cultures: the health professional's own culture, the patient's culture and the culture of the health system or institution.[2]

For some overseas-trained health professionals who come to countries such as Australia and work with Aboriginal people, there may be multiple cultural 'domains' to negotiate.[3] There is the dominant culture of the country, which will determine the paradigm and world view of the health culture, and there will be the culture of the patients, which may be completely different again. Similarly, when a British or Australian doctor goes to work in Nepal there is the culture of the well-educated Indian and Nepalese doctors and the very different culture of the local people, who are extremely poor, have a different religion and certainly a different view of health. Defined components of transcultural counselling are shown in Box 8.1.

BOX 8.1 COMPONENTS OF TRANSCULTURAL COUNSELLING (ADAPTED FROM D'ARDENNE AND MAHTANI)[1]

- Sensitivity to cultural variation, including recognition of the therapist's own cultural bias and/or ethnocentrism.
- Knowledge relating to the cultural background of the patient.
- Ability and commitment to develop a therapeutic relationship that reflects the cultural needs of the patient.
- Skill in working with the increased complexity that transcultural counselling involves.

PRELIMINARY CONSIDERATIONS

Culture is expressed in how we communicate – be this verbally or non-verbally, consciously or subconsciously. Culture begins to affect behaviour before speech develops. It impacts on the very early development of the brain and how a person relates to themselves, other people, the world, their concept of God and their future. For those within the same culture, communication can be subtle, non-verbal and subconscious, maybe even intuitive. Communicating across cultures will mostly only be verbal and cannot transcend the consciousness of the two individuals. Only part of human communication is through speech, and so communicating across cultures is always going to be fraught with the difficulties inherent in missing the majority of the message. This is especially important in mental health, where the clinician is often attempting to help the patient have access to the unconscious driving forces that may be part of their illness. Errors in interpretation are likely to be common in the situation where the clinician is unaware of the limitations of relying only on verbal communication.

For example, in Western culture 'no' and 'yes' are used commonly as replies to questions but in many cultures there may be no words that can be interpreted as 'no' or 'yes' and responses will always be more expansive. 'No' may never be an appropriate direct response because of 'shame' or 'saving face' or 'politeness' and so a negative answer will never be given. Questions need to be phrased in a way that allows a more indirect response and the clinician needs to have a heightened awareness of what is really being said. The other problem is of course the hierarchical relationship that exists between doctor and patient in many cultures. Patients will want to 'please' the doctor and give the response that they think the doctor wants to hear rather than what is truly happening for them.

There will always be a power relationship between a health professional and a patient. The patient is the one who is ill and asking for help, the health professional is the one who is running the consultation. It is the responsibility of the health professional to take the patient's culture into account during the clinical encounter, not to expect that the patient will comply with the culture of the health professional or the society. The patient is the one who is the most vulnerable and usually presents with less personal or sometimes social resources for cultural change. For the patient, health is the main priority. During times of stress, patients will often lose more recent skills such as language and cultural nuances, which is likely to make it even more difficult to negotiate the consultation.

INTERPRETERS, ADVOCATES AND CULTURAL MENTORS

An experienced interpreter will be needed for most psychotherapy if the patient and health professional speak different languages. Interpreting in a mental health setting is an even more specialised skill than it is in other medical settings.

The patient's first language will be the one with which they have access to dreams, childhood memories, world view and many deeply held cultural beliefs. An interpreter will also get around the problem of the patient struggling to find words to explain feelings in a second language in a stressful situation, but the interpreter will often be left trying to translate culture-bound words.[4] Some issues are sacred or forbidden and will not be discussed with particular groups such as certain genders, language groupings, family members or religions. This might actually affect the choice of interpreter more than it affects the choice of health professional, as it is the interpreter who is the 'speaker of the language'. The stigma and shame associated with mental illness becomes a huge risk when a third party is involved, especially if the interpreter is from the same community as the patient.

Interpreting unique cultural ideas, psychological concepts, feelings and vague thoughts will be difficult from both sides. Interpreters need to provide an interpretation as equivalent in meaning and connotation as possible; however, some words and phrases may have no direct translation and the interpreter may speak the language but may miss some of the subtle cultural meanings. Interpreters ideally should have relevant cultural knowledge and appropriate professional backgrounds.[5] Thus employing a family member as an interpreter is not recommended, though often this is an expedient solution to the problem of finding a suitable professional. Literal translation is appropriate if the patient's speech is confused or incoherent because there is thought disorder, flight of ideas or dysphasia. Interpreters will also come with their own backgrounds and opinions, and discomfort, fear or a judgemental attitude of the interpreter are likely to adversely affect the interview. Whenever possible, the same interpreter should be used in each consultation for a patient with mental health issues, as the patient needs to learn to feel comfortable with the interpreter as well as the therapist.

Often the only available interpreter is a family member or friend. There are many problems with using family members and friends as interpreters. They cannot be expected to know medical terminology, might filter information, are not bound by rules of ethics or confidentiality, and might not be able to handle or cope with things they hear. Sensitive issues such as sexual problems, mental health issues or domestic violence are unlikely to be discussed where a family member is interpreting. Health professionals risk a compromised quality of care and the potential to commit serious errors if a family member or friend is used. In addition, our legal colleagues constantly remind us of the importance of confidentiality, fully informed consent and a thorough understanding of illnesses and their management for all patients.

Patient advocates have different roles, working on behalf of patients to ensure that care is optimal and that there is good communication and shared understanding between the patient and health professionals. An advocate should not make decisions for a patient or express views as to which treatment option is best. Advocates should not have access to a patient's medical records and must be aware of their obligation to respect patient confidentiality. Health advocacy, as opposed to straightforward interpretation, may provide a useful way of bridging gaps in cultural understanding.

Cultural mentors are also important as links between patient, community and health professional. The role and scope of cultural mentoring is discussed in Chapter 2.

BOX 8.2 CASE STUDY 1 (AYEN'S STORY)

Ayen came from the desert in Sudan. She had never learnt to read or write and came to see the doctor because she had some 'women's problems'. There was no female Nuer interpreter so there was a Nuer to Sudanese Arabic interpreter and a Sudanese Arabic to English interpreter. Ayen came with her own adult daughter and niece. All five of the Sudanese women were very tall and were dressed in brightly coloured traditional dress. The doctor was short and blonde of Anglo-Scandinavian background.

First the doctor asked Ayen how long she had been here, where she had come from, where she was born, who in her family were here, who had been left behind, what she thought of the food and the housing in Australia etc. Everything was translated into Sudanese Arabic, then Nuer and then the reply translated back again.

The doctor then opened the patient's file and looked at her date of birth. 'Goodness', she said, 'You're 70!! I hope I look like you when I'm 70'. This was translated to Sudanese Arabic and Nuer. The patient replied and the other three Nuer-speaking women roared with laughter. Finally containing themselves, the reply was translated into Sudanese Arabic. She too, laughed long and loud. The doctor was enjoying being part of so much laughter with a group of women but was a bit concerned about what she had said that had caused so much frivolity.

At last the reply was interpreted into English. Ayen said 'I'm very sorry doctor but you're never going to look like me!!'

In that moment of shared humour, cultural and language differences disappeared.

THE INITIAL CONSULTATION

People take into account various factors when deciding whether to seek professional help about a healthcare concern. These will vary partly according to whether the patient has to pay for a consultation, the distance to travel plus the ease of access to a healthcare provider. Taken into account are the severity and effects of any symptoms, whether treatment such as drugs might be needed and the person's previous experience of healthcare interactions. Friends and family may also be consulted about the necessity to seek help.

When patients do decide to see a doctor they will have a problem, symptom or concern that they would like to discuss. This may be vague or well defined. Patients may have an idea of what the cause of the 'complaint' may be; they may have discussed the symptom with friends or family and have their opinions on diagnosis. They may have decided what they would like the doctor to do to resolve the problem, or they may have no particular expectations other than 'to get better'. All of these possible thoughts will be influenced by the person's psychosocial background, including cultural practices and beliefs.

Patients may choose their general practice on the basis of the attributes of the doctors and primary healthcare team. For example, they may wish to have the choice of female or male doctor, or they may seek out a nurse who speaks their first language. In some areas they may not have such a choice, or when they attend the practice the person they prefer to see may not be available. A difficult issue is whether a patient should be able to decline to see a particular professional on the basis of ethnicity, as it would not be considered good practice if a doctor refused to see a patient because of ethnicity alone. The General Medical Council's guidelines on personal beliefs and the doctor–patient relationship address the issues of how beliefs, including religious beliefs, must not be allowed to affect the professional judgement of a doctor, which should be based only on their clinical knowledge.[6]

The initial contact between a 'new' patient and the doctor will almost always involve an unconscious judgement on both sides based on appearance, including age, gender and dress. Such judgement may even have started before visual contact, through name alone. The patient may have been recommended to this doctor and therefore have some preconceived notions about quality and professionalism. If the patient is black, for example, and the doctor white, the doctor may choose to be 'colour blind' and ignore potential ethnic differences, not eluding to them in the course of the interaction. This course of action may be chosen to ensure that there is no overt racism in the consultation; however, in certain circumstances, the patient's ethnicity may have a bearing on the problem and may need to be acknowledged. If miscommunication occurs during the consultation, the doctor should raise the issue of potential barriers to the interaction, one of which may involve cultural ignorance or prejudice.

As with any consultation, introductions are important. Both parties may need to explain how their surname/family name is pronounced and mention how they wish to be addressed. The doctor should also stress that anything discussed in the consultation is confidential, as this may not be known to a patient coming from a different health system or culture. If an interpreter is being used, it is also important to stress that the interpreter is also bound to confidentiality. This is particularly important when patient and interpreter come from a small community within the dominant culture.

The doctor normally begins a consultation, after appropriate introductions, with an invitation to the patient to 'present the problem'.[1] Sometimes the patient will give a clear indication of what this is: 'I have a pain in my side',

'I am worried about losing weight', 'I cannot sleep'. Of course this 'presenting complaint' may or may not be the patient's main concern. There are cultural and social determinants of what patients believe a doctor is for and what the doctor can do. In the UK, where a patient can see a GP free at the point of service, patients feel able to discuss housing problems and domestic issues straight out. This may seem unusual behaviour to doctors from other countries. Conversely, patients from outside the UK may feel the need to give the doctor a physical symptom before being invited to explore more psychosocial concerns. Thus the presenting complaint may not be clear or agreed between the two parties.

BOX 8.3 FACTORS POTENTIALLY RELEVANT
TO THE PSYCHOSOCIAL HISTORY

- Identification with ethnicity (a third-generation Briton of Indian descent may identify with both cultures socially but with Asian ethnicity).
- Where born and raised (need to be careful not to assume that patients were not born in the country where consultation is taking place).
- Citizen of which country (this may have implications for funding of healthcare interaction).
- Support networks (particularly important if moved countries, as may be sparse).
- Family and friends (as with support networks).
- Does the patient/client see culture or ethnicity as part of the problem?

The patient-centred approach to interaction includes an exploration of the patient's ideas, concerns and expectations. To these should be added a sensitive elicitation of the patient's religious, cultural and family background and value system as appropriate (Box 8.3). The doctor should acknowledge that the patient may not be used to discussing sensitive and personal issues with a health professional. For example, the doctor may say: 'I can understand and appreciate that you might be finding it very difficult to talk about your problems with a stranger. How do you feel about it? Who do you usually confide in?' Other questions that might be considered in consultations with patients from other countries are shown in Box 8.4 (a fuller list is given in the Cultural Awareness Tool – Chapter 2, Box 2.2).

BOX 8.4 QUESTIONS TO CONSIDER ASKING PATIENTS FROM OTHER COUNTRIES

- What do you think these symptoms would mean in X? *(insert name of patient's country).*
- If you consulted a doctor/healer with these symptoms in X, what would you expect to happen/be the outcome?
- What would you do if you had these symptoms in X?

Difficulties may also arise if the patient is from the dominant culture and the doctor/health professional is not (or perceived not to be). If there appears to be discomfort (and if the doctor feels uncomfortable, this may be a mirror of the patient's feelings), the doctor could say: 'Are you finding it difficult to talk about your problems with me because I am male/female/from a different cultural background and/or religion?'

Patients prejudge doctors as much as the other way round. A doctor of Asian ancestry may be assumed to be from another country whereas he was born and educated within the UK. A white doctor may have been born and educated in Eastern Europe. Following a highly publicised case of professional misconduct in Australia relating to an international medical graduate from India, many Australians did not wish to consult with doctors who appeared to be from the same Indian background as that doctor, though many of these professionals were Australian.

THE PATIENT–PROFESSIONAL INTERACTION

The success of the interaction partly relates to the extent of the doctor's knowledge about the patient's cultural background and to the extent of the patient's knowledge about the doctor's cultural background, as well as to knowledge about the health system on both sides. Medical jargon, difficult for people to understand at the best of times, will be even more obstructive if the doctor, the patient or even both parties do not have English as a first language. The doctor should be constantly checking for verbal and non-verbal cues that suggest a lack of understanding. If the patient perceives that the doctor is not able to understand the interaction or misinterprets this as annoyance or time pressure, the patient may become silent and acquiescent. Summarising at intervals allows checking for understanding on both sides. Both doctor and patient should summarise as appropriate.

When working with patients we constantly use verbal and non-verbal cues to assess how the consultation is progressing. Such cues may not be interpreted correctly on either side in transcultural interactions. There are cultural differences in eye contact and gazing behaviour, what is seen as personal space, how the body is orientated, what is acceptable in terms of physical contact and displays of emotion.[7] The doctor should check by asking 'How does that make you feel?', 'How are you feeling?' or 'Can I check if this is making you upset or unhappy?', for example. The doctor may also need to signpost her own emotions: 'This is a difficult area for me to explore as I feel I am upsetting you – is it all right to continue?'

Open questions will be of most use when eliciting the patient's expectations rather than giving him a menu of options to choose from. However, if the expectations are unrealistic or cannot be met at the time, the doctor may need to explain the options after this initial scoping.

Considerations to be kept in mind during transcultural interactions are shown in Box 8.5.

BOX 8.5 TRANSCULTURAL INTERACTIONS – BEAR THESE IN MIND

- Be careful of the assumption that a patient's problems are related to their cultural experience or background.
- However, the patient's relationship to his/her culture(s) needs to be considered and explored as appropriate.
- As with all consultations, flexibility, openness to experience and empathy are required.
- Each patient is unique but similar to other human beings in biological and psychosocial terms – be careful of stereotyping or prejudging.
- Try to consult holistically – taking account of the whole person rather than the symptoms presented.

SETTING BOUNDARIES

Patients and professionals working within new health systems may have different expectations of each other's role. This is often the case with counsellors or with counselling sessions. The patient should be aware of how to access the health system and the counsellor. The patient should also be aware of which health professional is responsible for what. If the patient is seeing a counsellor or therapist but has a concurrent physical problem, he should know that he can still see his GP. If the GP is providing counselling sessions, which will be longer consultations than normal, the patient should be aware that these sessions are not for other problems. (Of course splitting interactions in this way is not particularly holistic but is necessary in some circumstances. For example, a patient who requires a repeat prescription for diabetes and a check-up should not usually expect this during a counselling consultation.) The professional and patient need to agree on the length of consultations, how often they will take place and what should happen in between consultations if there are major problems.

The seating arrangements need to be agreed, and whether the doctor/counsellor can access a computer during the consultation. The issue of physical contact should be explored or intuited – a doctor who is used to holding a stressed patient's hand may need to rethink this strategy with certain patients or discuss whether it is acceptable.

In counselling sessions, the counsellor expects the patient to open up about very personal issues and is likely to explore family and intimate relationships. However, the counsellor will not expect to discuss their own personal details with the patient. The flow of information is usually in one direction. GPs, however, may expect some questions about family if they have photographs of children or partners on their desks. How far to 'allow' personal questions is a difficult decision and depends very much on the circumstances and purpose of the interaction.

Ethical problems may arise during consultations, particularly in relation to boundary setting but also in relation to confidentiality and disclosure by the patient of racism within other healthcare settings. Some of the problems may occur because of cultural differences in values, leading to a cultural conflict. To resolve such conflicts four steps may be taken.[8] Of course the first step is to try to prevent such conflicts. This is possible through adequate learning and the development of sensitivity. Secondly, health professionals should not blame patients or themselves for conflicts but rather define the conflict contextually so that everyone may help to resolve the problem. Thirdly, solutions should be suggested that are in line with defined management goals. Lastly, the professional should discuss the problem openly, seek clarification and acknowledge any issues relating to cultural differences arising in the consultations.

STANDARD PHYSICAL AND MENTAL HEALTH QUESTIONNAIRES

Some GPs and therapists like to use questionnaires to assess the extent of their patients' problems. There are many such rating scales for conditions ranging from disability to depression.[9] Such instruments may have not been validated for people from the non-dominant culture and should be used with caution.

However, there are several screening tools that have been validated for use in specific cultures, usually as a self-assessment tool or to be read directly to the patient by someone from the same language group. Scales such as the General Health Questionnaire (GHQ), the Hopkins Symptom Checklist (HSCL-25) and the Personal Health Questionnaire (PHQ) have been validated for use in many different countries, and some for specific minority groups such as people of Pakistani or Indian origin in the UK.[10,11]

The validation process is complex and involves translation from English and then translation back into English by different translators. The tool is then tested on a group of people and a diagnosis made by qualified mental health professionals. The 'cut-off' point for what is deemed to be a diagnosis or 'case' using the assessment tool can then be validated for that particular group of people using that translation. Most tools aim to assess patients over a specified period of time such as the 'past few weeks' and have a Likert scale or similar that gives a range of options gauging change in function or level of distress.[12] Hence using an assessment tool translated by an interpreter in a one-to-one situation is not a valid way of using any of the tools.

The desire for a standardised assessment tool stems from an 'etic' (*see* Chapter 9, Box 9.6) opinion of mental illness. Use of a screening tool implies that there is a set of universal symptoms that can be used in any culture to identify depression, anxiety, PTSD or other mental health problems. The 'emic' view would be that each culture will present differently and that a tool that will pick up mental illness in a variety of cultures is not possible. A 'middle ground' is the rigorous validation that has been applied to some tools, with modifications such as a change in the 'cut-off point' for saying what is and isn't likely to be mental illness in that culture. Recognition of other variations such as with different genders can be accounted for, but differences with self-administration versus being read to and the environment in which the tool is administered cannot be predicted accurately. Patients with mental illness in cultures without a mental health tradition are unlikely to score above the threshold for a 'case' using tools that have a large number of mood questions, but they may score more highly on tools that emphasise somatic symptoms.[13]

Despite being validated, screening tools may still result in faulty diagnoses, as they will not be able to sample the culturally specific symptoms and ways of expressing distress. They may not be truly equivalent in areas such as the linguistic (the same word will have a different meaning), conceptual (concepts such as dependency or sadness will have different connotations), scale (e.g. true and false, Likert scales are unfamiliar) or normative (normal is very culturally mediated).[12] Tools that rely on 'true/false' answers will not be useful in some cultures, as it may be impolite to say that something is false or there may not be a dedicated word for false. There are likely to be many other reasons for an assessment tool being difficult to interpret in other cultures. For example, in some cultures it would be seen as disrespectful not to worry about relatives who were sick or unsafe. To say that you had 'lost much sleep over worry' (GHQ) would mean that you are a good relative.

The other argument against screening tools is that they do not assess the difference between a normal response to severe personal or environmental stress and an abnormal response to minor stress. Indeed this brings the discussion back to whether the Western world is considering a reaction to such socioenvironmental circumstances as extreme poverty, torture or trauma as 'normal' or as mental illnesses needing 'treatment'. What is 'normal' and 'expected' in a situation is very culturally, socially and sometimes politically mediated, and so what is an 'abnormal' or 'traumatic' experience will similarly be different in each culture. Part of the validation process for a tool should include an investigation of what is deemed to be pathology by the society in which the tool is to be used.

The use of a screening tool implies that a 'diagnosis' can be made of a mental health disorder. However, most of the tools will be picking up psychological distress and it is important not to immediately jump to the conclusion that the patient needs or wants treatment in the Western sense. When working with refugees for instance, the pathologising of the reaction to torture as PTSD is seen by some as a way of downplaying the significance of the torture as a political tool aiming to destroy a person's attachment to their own integrity, reality, spirituality and hope.

Whatever tool is used in clinical practice, it is only useful if it is interpreted by someone with the skills, time and resources to deal with the results that have been found. Screening tools are not a substitute for clinical expertise and should only be used in an environment where a health professional is able to go through the questions with the patient and then help implement management and a safety plan if necessary.

PATIENT PARTNERSHIP

The patient-centred model combined with the concept of patient partnership may be used in Western consultations. This model may not be the most appropriate in the transcultural setting, when patients may not wish to make decisions with the doctor without involving family. The non-directive counselling model may also be difficult to enact if the patient wishes to be directed as to what to do next. Of course GPs and other health professionals do not always share decisions and sometimes are more directive than would occur within a 'counselling interaction'. Patients may not be aware of the different types of management styles depending on the professional, the nature of the interaction and their own problem. Seeing one doctor who says 'You must take this medication' and then a therapist who asks 'What do you think is the best way forward?' may be confusing.

The best approach would seem to be to decide jointly on therapeutic goals (though families may be involved in this decision). A consensus on management is more likely to succeed.

REFLECTION ON THE CONSULTATION

Transcultural interactions are often difficult and professionals may wish to reflect on them in order to improve skills in these consultations. Box 8.6 includes trigger questions for reflection both pre and post consultations. In practices where many transcultural interactions occur, such questions could form the basis of an educational session.

BOX 8.6 TRIGGER QUESTIONS FOR REFLECTION

- What do I define as my own cultural identity?
- What has influenced my cultural identity and how was it formed?
- How do I/did I feel after the consultation and why?
- In what ways did the transcultural nature of the consultation affect my performance?
- Was I aware of cultural differences?
- Should I have been?
- Did I explore relevant lifestyle factors?
- Did I consider cultural factors in the problems presented?
- Might racism be an issue for this patient? How would I know?
- Might my prejudices have affected the interaction?
- Might the patient's prejudices have affected the interaction?
- Does the patient understand my culture and/or the culture of the practice?
- What do I need to do/read/practise in order to improve my performance?
- How could I be better prepared to interact with this patient again?
- How could I get feedback from this patient about the interaction?
- What do/would my colleagues think about this interaction?
- Does this consultation reflect in any way on my own experience of transcultural interactions when I am not working in my professional capacity?

Reflection and peer discussion can be helped by videotaping consultations and watching them to gain feedback. However, such taping may not be acceptable to some patients, even with explanation of the educational purpose of the taping.

We may find it difficult to appreciate just how closely our cultural upbringing influences us, especially if we have trained and work within the same culture. Our everyday experience impinges on our attitudes and values without our awareness. Moving to another culture shows us the effects of culture shock (*see* Chapter 7 and 11) and how much our professional identity is bound up with our cultural heritage. Trying to immerse oneself in another culture, either through moving country or interacting transculturally, is similar to trying to think in a foreign language when we only know its basics. It is tiring.

Reading books about other cultures helps us to understand the social and psychological background of our patients. Knowledge of the history and political milieu of countries from which our patients come is also helpful. Textbooks with cultural menus (e.g. what form of contraception is acceptable to which religion, who eats what foods etc) are helpful but lack the richness and variation of cultural life. We need to be careful of stereotyping. A patient may not identify with what we presume is their 'obvious' group, or they may describe themselves in terms of the group identity but express their lifestyle in a personal way.

PATTERNS OF CULTURAL DIFFERENCES

Six fundamental patterns of cultural differences have been recognised by workers in this field (Box 8.7).[14] Communication (verbal and non-verbal) is an obvious area, as is mentioned repeatedly in this book. Ways of dealing with conflict vary from the direct approach common in many Western societies to the more discrete model of Eastern cultures, where 'saving face' is important. Some cultures prefer decisions to be made by group or family discussion, whereas in others decision-making is an individual responsibility relating to hierarchy and position. Ways of expressing emotions vary from frank displays of crying and laughing to discrete or even neutral changes in body language. The Western scientific tradition places great stress on measuring, counting and statistics in the quest for knowledge. Compare this to the more spiritual or intuitive way found in other communities. Of course these differences are generalisations and should be treated as guides only.

<hr>

BOX 8.7 PATTERNS OF CULTURAL DIFFERENCES[14]

<hr>

- Communication styles.
- Attitudes towards conflict.
- Approaches to completing tasks.
- Decision-making styles.
- Attitudes towards disclosure.
- Approaches to knowing.

CONCEPTS OF THE SELF: INDIVIDUALISM AND COLLECTIVISM

One aspect of cultural diversity or difference that is often discussed when considering a person's world view is the concept of individualism as compared to collectivism. Cultural descriptions tend to focus on difference, while cultural diversity literature focuses on valuing such difference. In the one-to-one setting of many patient–health professional interactions, how important is the distinction between those cultures that are identified as individualistic and those as collectivist, and what practical value does such distinction have?

While the notion of a private inner self is probably universal, the description of its exact content and structure differs markedly between cultures.[15] This will affect the way an individual expresses their thought processes, emotions and relationships, and will influence any mental pathology. For instance,

> The Western experience with depressive disorders may be a function of Western preoccupation with guilt, individualism, self-structure, self-control, personal responsibility, and an 'abstract' language structure that creates distance between the person and his or her experience through language and self. In contrast the Eastern experience of depression tends to reflect the integrated conception of mind and body as one and is portrayed through somatic symptoms rather than feelings of sadness.[16]

Carl Rogers, the originator of client-centred counselling, defined the concept of the self as: 'composed of such elements as the perceptions of one's characteristics and abilities; the percepts and concepts of self in relation to others and the environment; the value qualities which are perceived as associated with experiences and objects; and goals and ideas which are perceived as having positive and negative valences' (p. 51).[17] Self-concept is in the cognitive or thinking domain, in contrast to self-esteem, which is in the affective or feeling domain. Rogers' system of psychotherapy was built upon the premise of the importance of the self and the need for self-awareness.

The independent self may also be characterised as a self-contained, individuated, separated identity defined by clear boundaries from others; the individual is a separate and autonomous entity comprising distinct attributes which in turn cause behaviour.[15] A healthy self is defined as one that can maintain integrity and clear boundaries across diverse social environments, that can differentiate itself from significant others as part of the maturation process and that can successfully fend off challenge from others.

Many commentators believe that such concepts of self are mainly situated in the Western individualistic tradition, in contrast to the Eastern more collectivist world view. The Western 'self' is an egocentric person set apart from others, whereas in Eastern sociocentric communities there is a greater connection of the self to family, friends and the community,[18] with an emphasis on fitting in and harmonious interdependence.[15] 'Moreover, sociocentric selves are primarily based on bonds, allegiances and commitments to persons, families, and communities; individualistic selves are marked by the unique attributes harboured by and within the person. The selves of specific persons are anchored between these two reference points' (p. 27).[18]

The theory of the individualistic-collectivist axis has generated a great deal of discussion and research amongst psychologists. The simple heuristic that West equals self/personal and East equals group/community, while helpful to some extent, cannot be relied upon in interactions with patients. Again it is important to avoid stereotyping. Box 8.8 lists some of the attributes of individualism and collectivism. Individualists are thought to thrive in impersonal social and work settings but are vulnerable to loneliness; collectivists work well in small teams but may feel stifled in that they have to ignore personal ambitions.

BOX 8.8 BROAD DISTINCTIONS BETWEEN
INDIVIDUALISM AND COLLECTIVISM

Individualism
'Western'
Interpersonal ties are loose
Responsibility often only extends to self or immediate family
Relationships – small number but intense
Personal ambition is important
Loyalty may shift
Consumerism
Tends to be secular

Usually assumes people are responsible for their own misfortune
Right to privacy
Pleasure-seeking and self-fulfillment
Financial security
Freedom of choice
Status is defined by achievements
Relationships mostly horizontal and equal

Collectivism
Indigenous cultures and much of the developing world
Spirituality pervades every aspect of lives of people from most indigenous
  cultures and cannot be differentiated from either their physical or mental
  well-being
Ecological
Consensual and communal
Social harmony more important than individual interests
Fatalistic, favour concession and compromise
Duties and obligations
Tend to be vertical relationships based on unequal power
Strong interpersonal ties
Responsibility to extended family greater than that to self
Relationships – multiple
Personal ambition is secondary to well-being of group
Groups are strong and cohesive and often lifelong
Loyalty has to be unquestioning
View illness as usually imposed on an individual by an outside agency

It is important to realise that the distinctions as listed do not mean that there is no sense of the individual in collectivist societies. A more unifying theory of self has been proposed that defines self-concept as including both elements of personal identity and group identity, such that individuality is present in all cultures, whereas individualism as a particular form of individuality is a marker of Western developed societies.[19] Everyone demonstrates aspects of self-esteem and group-esteem, and these should be seen as complementary assets rather than being in competition.[19] Patients from Western backgrounds who appear to espouse individualism may well belong to many social, political and/or religious groups with whom they feel an affinity. A certain amount of self-esteem is required in a collectivist society so that a person is of value to the group and carries out group tasks with commitment.

In transcultural interactions the professional needs to be aware that a practical outcome of the self versus group dichotomy is that the expectation of patients may be different. A person from a Western culture may see the best outcome as personal growth, self-actualisation or satisfaction, 'finding oneself', whereas the person from a collectivist culture may see the best outcome as that benefiting his community/group, which may not be necessarily the best for himself. Note, however, that the notion of the possibility of personal growth or development as a goal of treatment has been eschewed by the narrative therapy school. In this approach humans are not thought of as having universal inner essences or one human nature unrelated to cultural and life experiences. Narrative therapy helps people reassess their life stories and facilitates them finding realistic solutions to their problems[20] (*see also* Chapter 5).

CONFIDENTIALITY

The Western culture of individuality favours a strong ethical principle of confidentiality. The information about the patient's life and health belongs to that patient and consent must be gained for the information to be shared, even with close members of the family. An adult patient is expected to speak on their own behalf and to ask their own questions.

This is not the case in many cultures. For those more sociocentric cultures where the self-other boundary is not so firm, it is not seen as a breach of confidentiality if specified members of the family are privy to information. They may be involved in the consultation from the outset, speak for the patient, ask questions, expect to be informed of the results of investigations and be part of any management planning. In some cultures the specified member or members of the family may not be the mother or father, as expected in a Western culture, but may be the grandmother, an uncle, a niece or the eldest son. In many countries where lives are lived very close to each other and medical care is disorganised or under-resourced, confidentiality is a luxury or is not possible.

BOX 8.9 CASE STUDY 2 (AYAN AND XUE'S STORIES)

Ayan is a 35-year-old female refugee from Somalia who is living in the East End of London in a hostel. She is married with two children aged five and three. She comes to the local GP surgery with her husband, Abdi. She has only a few words of English but her husband, who was a business student in his native country, has a reasonable command of the language. Abdi has been looking for a job and spends most of his time away from the hostel. Abdi explains that his wife has back pain and is always tired. She finds it difficult to look after the children and is hardly eating. She wants to sleep all the time. Abdi says he is also concerned that his wife has not become pregnant again though they have not been using contraception for some time.

Xue is a 25-year-old physics student from China. She sees a GP at the university health centre because she has developed a rash on her face in the last few weeks. Her English is fairly good but she is not familiar with medical terminology. To the GP the rash is obviously acne and Xue knows this word. She accepts a prescription for a cream but seems unsatisfied with the consultation. However, the doctor decides not to pursue this as she is running late that morning. Xue returns a week later as her face is no better. The GP explains that the cream will take several weeks to work. She asks Xue what is bothering her. Xue explains that she does not think the problem can be acne as she never had the condition as a teenager. Moreover, her flatmates, who are Polish and English, have told her that she would feel better if she started having sex. Xue has promised her parents she will remain a virgin until she marries but now she is concerned that her skin is reacting to her lifestyle. Her friends have no problems with their skin and they regularly sleep with their boyfriends. The doctor spends some time talking through this 'culture clash' but when Xue asks if there are any tablets she could take, the doctor advises the contraceptive pill (a particular formulation that is licensed for the treatment of acne). Xue becomes even more confused and begins to stay at home more because she is embarrassed about the way she looks.

Ayan and Xue are under tremendous stress. A health professional who is consulted by either woman may feel overwhelmed by the enormity of the task in understanding their personal histories. How is Ayan's GP to untangle her story with the barriers of both language and culture? Moreover, it is likely that her husband and children are also suffering. Ayan's symptoms may be due to both physical and psychological causes. Unravelling the aetiology and then instituting a culturally sensitive and realistic management plan is going to take a lot of effort and time. Xue's problem appears simple at the start. The GP interacts with her the way she would with her native-born patients. Many young women are now aware that the pill may be used to treat acne – though of course others are not. It is important not to make assumptions about any patient, but with Xue the doctor has the added problem of miscommunication and unless she is prepared to spend time on her explanations, Xue is likely to become more stressed. A well-meaning doctor, with other patients like these, is going to become frustrated and possibly therefore lose empathy over time.

Not only are these people undergoing culture shock and failing to adapt to their new environments, they may have mental health problems relating to their life circumstances prior to the move. Trying to sort out the immediate maladaptation may not help in the long run.

PRACTICAL POINTS

➤ How and what a person presents to a health professional will be influenced by the person's psychosocial background, including cultural practices and beliefs.

➤ The initial contact between a 'new' patient and the doctor will almost always involve a judgement on both sides based on appearance, including age, gender and dress.

➤ As well as exploring a patient's ideas, concerns and expectations, the health professionals should sensitively explore the patient's religious, cultural and family background and value system as appropriate.

➤ Knowledge of the history and political milieu of countries from which our patients come is helpful.

➤ The Western culture of individuality favours a strong ethical principle of confidentiality but this principle may need to be adapted for collectivist societies.

➤ Interpreting in a mental health setting is an even more specialised skill than it is in other medical settings.

REFERENCES

1 D'Ardenne P, Mahtani A. *Transcultural Counselling in Action*. 2nd ed. London: Sage; 1999.
2 Kagawa-Singer M, Kassim-Lakha S. A strategy to reduce cross-cultural miscommunication and increase the likelihood of improving health outcomes. *Acad Med.* 2003; 78: 577–87.
3 Arkles R. *Overseas Trained Doctors in Aboriginal and Torres Strait Islander Health Services: a literature review*. Muru Marri Indigenous Health Unit and the Cooperative Research Centre for Aboriginal Health; 2006. Available at: www.crcah.org.au/publications/downloads/Overseas-Trained-Doctors.pdf (accessed January 2008).
4 Tamasese K, Peteru C, Waldegrave C, *et al*. Ole Taeao Afua, the new morning: a qualitative investigation into Samoan perspectives on mental health and culturally appropriate services. *Aust N Z J Psychiatry*. 2005; 39: 300–9.
5 Robinson L. Intercultural communication in a therapeutic setting. In: Coker N, editor. *Racism in Medicine*. London: King's Fund; 2001. pp. 191–210.
6 General Medical Council. *Personal Beliefs and Medical Practice*. London: GMC; 2008. Available at: www.gmcuk.org/guidance/ethical_guidance/personal_beliefs/personal_beliefs.asp (accessed April 2008).
7 Rozelle RM, Druckman D, Baxter JC. Non-verbal behaviour as communication. In: Hargie ODW, editor. *The Handbook of Communication Skills*. 2nd ed. London: Routledge; 1997.

8 Ridley CR, Liddle MC, Hill CL, *et al.* Ethical decision making in multicultural counseling. In: Ponterotto JG, Casas JM, Suzuki LA, *et al.*, editors. *Handbook of Multicultural Counselling.* 2nd ed. London: Sage; 2001. pp. 165–88.

9 McDowell I. *Measuring Health: A Guide to Rating Scales and Questionnaires.* 3rd ed. Oxford: Oxford University Press; 2006.

10 Husain N, Waheed W, Tomenson B, *et al.* The validation of personal health questionnaire amongst people of Pakistani family origin living in the United Kingdom. *J Affect Disord.* 2007; 97: 261–4.

11 Jacob K, Bhugra D, Mann A. The validation of the 12-item general health questionnaire among ethnic Indian women living in the United Kingdom. *Psychol Med.* 1997; 27: 1215–7.

12 Marsella A, Kaplan A, Suarez E. Cultural considerations for understanding, assessing, and treating depressive experience and disorder. In: Reinecke M, Davison M, editors. *Comparative Treatments of Depression.* New York: Springer Series on Comparative Treatments for Psychological Disorders; 2002. pp. 47–78.

13 Ventevogel P, De Vries G, Scholte W, *et al.* Properties of the Hopkins Symptom Checklist-25 (HSCL-25) and the Self-Reporting Questionnaire (SRQ-20) as screening instruments used in primary care in Afghanistan. *Soc Psychiatry Psychiatr Epidemiol.* 2007; 42: 328–35.

14 DuPraw ME, Axner M. *Working on Common Cross-Cultural Communications Challenges.* Available at: www.wwcd.org/action/ampu/crosscult.html#PATTERNS (accessed March 2008).

15 Markus HR, Kitayama S. Culture and the self: implications for cognition, emotion and motivation. *Psychol Rev.* 1991; 98: 224–53.

16 Marsella A. Culture and psychopathology. In: Kitayama S, Cohen D, editors. *Handbook of Cultural Psychology.* New York, Guilford Publications, Inc; 2007. pp. 797–818.

17 Rogers C. *Client-Centered Therapy: its current practice, implications and theory.* London: Constable; 1951.

18 Draguns JG. Universal and cultural threads in counselling individuals. In: Pedersen PB, Draguns JG, Lonner WJ, *et al.*, editors. *Counseling Across Cultures.* 6th ed. Los Angeles: Sage; 2008. pp. 21–36.

19 Cross Jnr WE, Cross TB. The big picture. Theorizing self-concept structure and construal. In: Pedersen PB, Draguns JG, Lonner WJ, *et al.*, editors. *Counseling Across Cultures.* 6th ed. Los Angeles: Sage; 2008. pp. 73–88.

20 Payne M. *Narrative Therapy.* 2nd ed. London: Sage; 2006.

9

Basic neuropsychiatry and the quest for normality

This chapter explores:
- Holism and dualism
- Physical changes in mental illness
- Sharing of information
- Definitions of normality
- The *Diagnostic and Statistical Manual of Mental Disorders* (DSM-IV)
- The International Guidelines for Diagnostic Assessment (IGDA)
- The healing art

Mind, body and soul: modern orthodox Western medicine both separates and brings together these three concepts. It separates because there are specialities devoted to neurology and the nervous system (the body), while psychiatry focuses on mental health and illness (the mind) or what lay people may call 'nerves'. The soul is rarely mentioned. Western medicine tends to adopt the Cartesian dualism approach attributed to Descartes (1596–1650), the concept of which originates from the Greek philosophers Plato and Aristotle. Plato stated that the source of intelligence could not be identified within the physical body, believing that the mind is non-physical. Descartes argued further that the mind is different from the brain thus leading to the idea of mind/ body dualism. Thus we have physicians for the body and psychiatrists for the mind. The spiritual side of human beings is delegated to the priest, holy man or guru and is rarely ventured into by the health professional.

More recently, medicine is trying to bring the three together: there are general practitioners who take care of the whole person, adopting a holistic approach to healthcare. We recognise the effects of the mind on the body (psychosomatic illness or hypertension, for example) and the body on the mind (hallucinations). Holism means also acknowledging the soul and the spiritual beliefs of patients, taking these into account when diagnosing and treating.

Our language and our terminology also both separate and amalgamate. As students we are taught to assess a patient's symptoms in terms of the physical, psychological and social. Therefore, as students we think of these as separate components until we learn to describe illness in terms of the biopsychosocial. But does adding the three words together really lead to integration? The examination is still divided into 'physical' and 'mental state'. Yet we now have the specialty of neuropsychiatry: the field of exploring what effect the brain and its biochemistry have on behaviour, mood and cognition. Just as the lesions of multiple sclerosis may be mapped to the central nervous system, so doctors look for the signs of mental illnesses in the brain through imaging, electro-probing and response to mind-altering substances. Cognition is an abstract concept related to intelligence, meaning knowing, applying knowledge and processing information. Cognitive ability stems from the brain at either a conscious or unconscious level.

PHYSICAL OR PSYCHOLOGICAL?

BOX 9.1 CASE STUDY 1 (SARAH'S STORY)

Sarah, a 33-year-old teacher, is diagnosed with depression by her GP. She has feelings of emptiness and lack of self-esteem. Her physical symptoms include loss of appetite, poor sleep and shortened concentration span. She says she no longer finds enjoyment in her job, home or social life. In the last year her mother died from breast cancer, she split up from a relationship of eight years and she was passed over for promotion. Her doctor explains her illness in physical and psychological terms. Sarah has had a series of difficult events in her life and has not adjusted to her losses. She has felt both guilty and angry, feelings common in bereavement. She needs to talk about these feelings and the way they are affecting her physically and emotionally. The doctor also explains that depression is caused by a relative lack of the brain chemical serotonin. This cannot be measured by blood tests but the people who lack this chemical are similar to people who require thyroid hormone for an underactive thyroid gland. Sarah would benefit from an antidepressant that boosts serotonin levels (an SSRI, or selective serotonin reuptake inhibitor). Alternatively she might benefit from counselling or cognitive behavioural therapy. Sarah is unsure what treatment option to choose: is it better to think of her depression as a physical or psychological aberration?

Many patients would have no difficulty accepting the concepts as outlined to Sarah. They are rooted within the Western notion of illness; the treatment of mental health problems by counselling, drugs or both; and the strong health belief that happiness is affected by life events. Moreover, media reporting and pharmaceutical advertising have led to the widespread idea that unhappiness is also an illness that should be reported and treated. The line between depression (which is recognised as illness) and unhappiness (a state of mind) is blurring. If we could measure serotonin levels, we would have a diagnostic test more powerful than simply listening to the patient. Subjectivity and cultural bias would be eliminated. In reality though, what we are likely to find is that some people who perceive themselves as happy have low levels of serotonin and some people who describe themselves as depressed would have normal to high levels. Human behaviour, emotion and the response to events are conditioned by our experiences as well as our genetic heritage – the nature versus nurture debate. But language is also a powerful arbiter of diagnosis. The human condition is difficult to put into words . . . how do I know that when you are unhappy you are feeling the same emotions as I do when I am sad?

These are difficult philosophical questions and the answers are harder to find when we also take into account cultural, religious and social beliefs. Perhaps the end point in the brain is the same but the pathways are different. Before scientists were able to research the brain and its function, humans tried to make sense of illness by attributing symptoms and signs to various phenomena that have relationships to their environments and belief systems. And even with applied science and a better understanding of the brain, we still struggle to align our health beliefs with what the experts tell us is really going on inside our head. Often we choose to accept an 'unscientific' explanation for our problems because then we can also choose a treatment that suits us and our lifestyle. People in developed countries have a menu of options with a range of prices and often swap between medical systems such as orthodox, complementary, traditional and frank quackery (Box 9.2) depending on the problem (though even quackery is a matter of opinion and custom).

BOX 9.2 EXAMPLES OF VARIOUS TREATMENT OPTIONS FOR MENTAL HEALTH PROBLEMS AVAILABLE IN DEVELOPED COUNTRIES

- Counselling.
- Psychotherapy.
- Psychoanalysis.
- Cognitive behavioural therapy (CBT).

- Gestalt therapy.
- Hypnotherapy.
- Narrative therapy.
- Prescribed medication.
- Over the counter medication (e.g. St John's wort).
- Meditation.
- Homeopathy.
- Crystal therapy.
- Aura reading and adjustment.
- Exercise.

Doctors from other countries may have difficulty understanding this vast array of treatments and may not ask patients what therapies they have tried before seeking more orthodox help. This is important, as patients who choose alternative therapies as a first-line treatment are less likely to take prescribed medication such as antidepressants. This may be the case even though they are seeking medical help. Moreover, complementary therapies are not without risk,[1] may not list all the ingredients they contain and may interact with prescribed drugs. It is important to explore patient expectations of consultations.

PHYSICAL CHANGES IN MENTAL ILLNESS

In lay people's terms, mental health and therefore mental illness are functions of the mind, and the mind is physically located within the brain. The brain may be affected by changes elsewhere in the body mediated through chemicals which can alter such states as consciousness and cognition. Patients are well aware that alcohol and some drugs impair thought and often judgement.

In medical terms we can describe the brain's anatomy, physiology and biochemistry. These are of course inter-related and disruptions of any can cause physical and mental disturbances. At the cellular level neural impulses are mediated by brain neurotransmitters, and through manipulation of these changes in mood and cognition may be precipitated. Psychotropic drugs work at this level.

Nine of the main neurotransmitters working within the central nervous system and their actions are shown in Box 9.3. There are many other neuropeptides that exert their effects on neural cell function.

BOX 9.3 MAIN NEUROTRANSMITTERS AND ACTIONS

Name	Action
Acetylcholine	neuromodulator – arousal and reward, activates muscles
Adenosine	energy transfer; inhibitor – promotes sleep, suppresses arousal
Adrenaline	fight or flight – short-term stress reaction
Aspartate	excitatory, provides resistance to fatigue
Dopamine	behaviour, cognition, motor activity, sleep, mood, learning
GABA	excitatory or inhibitory, relaxant, anti-anxiety
Glutamate	excitatory, cognition – learning and memory
Noradrenaline	alertness and arousal
Serotonin	mood, state of mind

Nerve cells communicate with one another through impulses working across synapses, the gaps between the neurones. This transmission is mediated through the release of neurotransmitters, each of which works in very different ways. The chemicals attach to the recipient cell at very specific receptors. Expanding knowledge of brain biochemistry has prompted some experts to predict that in future patients with mental illnesses will be diagnosed as having specific neurobiological dysfunction, allowing accurate targeting of drug treatment. The effects of psychotropic drugs may be predicted by their chemical structure and then their actual effects monitored clinically. However, other treatments, such as meditation, which do not involve external agents, also appear to work through chemical mediation, highlighting the complexity of this subject.

Some people do not like to be thought of as just a large chemical laboratory with all emotion related to the action of molecules. They may ask where does God, the gods, the soul or the underlying personality with its experiences come into the equation. Should our bodies be viewed as solely mechanical? Does mood alter neurotransmission? Or does altered neurotransmission for other reasons alter mood? These are important questions, as patients' health beliefs arise from many sources, not only peer-referenced evidence, double-blind control trials and scientific reasoning.

NEURAL PATHWAYS AND RELATIONSHIPS

The history of medicine is littered with good ideas and theories, many of which have not stood the test of time, and some of which seem positively odd in the twenty-first century. The last century was a time of great discoveries in medical science but for part of the century there was a division between the science of the mind, as theorised by psychoanalysts such as Freud and Jung, and neuroscience, which looked to decipher mysteries through identifying neurotransmitters and neural pathways. Freud is remembered mainly for his description of the subconscious. His belief that children suppressed insatiable sexual desires and that discussing such repressed memories could help combat neuroses later in life is now largely discredited.

How memories are stored, accessed and often distorted from reality is now explained in terms of neural pathways and connections. Damage to certain areas of the brain and their neural connections has led to a greater understanding of what happens and where in neuroanatomical terms. In their book *A General Theory of Love*, three American psychiatrists write about the relationship between the limbic system in the brain and the neocortex.[2] The limbic system is seen as the processor and regulator of emotions. A healthy limbic system builds up the right connections during a healthy and happy childhood with the right amount of interdependence between child and parents. The child learns the basics of optimal relationships between humans and also those which may exist between humans and other animals. Through these relationships, neural pathways are created whose integrity is important for the pattern of subsequent relationships as the child matures and moves into adult life, looking for true love and often a lifelong bond with another.

The book does not dissect its thesis from any transcultural aspects. But when thinking culturally, the reader might consider how the pathways in the limbic system and their connections with the cortex may differ between societies with a strongly individualistic tendency, where extended families are not the norm and children are often cared for from outside the home in nurseries, and the collectivist cultures, where children are reared within the extended family. Derangements in family life caused by bereavement, wars, separation and/or divorce may lead to difficulties in relationships later in life – this seems a logical conclusion but in this book a neurological basis for such problems is eloquently argued.[2]

From birth we are programmed to have relationships. Bowlby's work with monkeys showed that babies learn quickly how to keep their mothers near them, as they are essential to their well-being. This is more than just about food and warmth. The closeness of the mother ensures that she can fulfil the baby's need for attachment and security. A baby who has had his or her 'inarticulate desires' met by his or her mother is likely to be a physically and mentally healthier adult.[2]

The genetic make-up of the brain is an unalterable template but the neurones are destroying and building new connections throughout life. Unused brain cells are 'pruned' and connections that are used more often are strengthened. After the initial accelerated brain growth before birth and in the first 18 months, there is a bout of pruning, and this happens again in the teenage years. These are times when the family, community and cultural environment is going to have a strong influence on what is deemed 'normal', 'good' and 'useful' by the brain. The brain becomes 'hardwired' with what is happening in the surroundings.[2]

SHARING OF INFORMATION

During patient–professional interactions we assume there is some common ground between the two people communicating. Sharing information is an important component of the consultation. The health professional elicits a history, gathering information from the patient and fitting it into a schema designed to produce a diagnosis or list of possible diagnoses (the differential diagnosis). This history (the patient's story) and the hypothesis relating to diagnosis ideally should be paraphrased in the health professional's words. This should then be fed back to the patient and agreement reached as to what has been said and understood. In the case of mental illness, the health professional may couch the explanation in terms of brain biochemistry or may use a more analytical framework ('I think your anxiety relates to the traumatic episode, your mugging, five years ago') or other frameworks such as behavioural or social. Of course we can never be completely sure of the accuracy of these cause and effect solutions. Explaining the neuropsychiatry of depression should take more than five minutes – how much detail is required? Does it matter how accurate or even truthful this exposition is, if the patient understands and this understanding aids treatment and recovery? Moreover, if during our careful eliciting of the story we have shown empathy towards the patient and gauged in what terms the patient is likely to want an explanation, then the content of the explanation may not be so important as the process of patient and health professional clarifying it together. However, this gauging relies on many cues, including cultural cues, and it is easy to get things wrong. Using certain words may raise the patient's anxiety rather than reducing it. One patient may be relieved to hear that her depression is due to a relative lack of serotonin, whereas another may prefer to think that his depression is due to his maladjustment to a new job, a process that takes time, whereas a chemical imbalance may sound permanent (and could be passed on to his children).

Health professionals often say that such and such feelings are normal in the circumstances. This is how other people feel. If they are normal, why do we suggest treating them? A patient relates new reactions to events to what has happened before – his normality. This feels different. Just what does this normal mean?

DEFINITIONS OF NORMALITY

Normal means lacking a significant deviation from the average. In mental health terms this raises the questions: what is average behaviour and what is significant? While a person may be labelled 'deviant', a pejorative term for someone behaving outside the accepted social norms, someone with odd behaviour who is considered harmless or even a figure of fun will be labelled 'eccentric'. Our language betrays our prejudices and stereotyping.

According to health statistics the majority of people in any country will suffer from a mental health problem during their lifetime. This of course depends on what a particular nation's doctors define as mental illness and what is perceived as normal, or in this context healthy, within a given society. History shows us that our definition of normal changes over time, being affected by biomedical research, society's evolution and even whims, philosophy and governments. To some people being viewed as 'normal' or accepted by the state and society is not something to be welcomed. But if we think of the opposite of normal as abnormal, this may be less acceptable a condition than, say, different or alternative, again highlighting the importance of language when discussing mental health.

It is easy to think of examples of how normal means various things to different people even within the same country, society and ethnic background. The work ethic of the generation who lived through the 1930s depression and World War II in the UK, now in their 80s, find it hard to understand the children of Generation X who are happy not to work, to dropout of society, to live on state handouts and sometimes to take drugs. To these octogenarians, who have worked all their lives, such behaviour is aberrant or abnormal. These elderly people are less likely to seek medical help for low mood or feel that it is a doctor's role to sort out the sorts of life problems that see their younger counterparts running to the surgery for pills for every ill.

In the last few decades new mental illnesses have been defined. To the cynic this often appears to happen when a new drug or a new indication for an old drug is available. A good example of this is categorisation of the fear that many of us have of speaking in public as social phobia. Of course the extent to which such fear disables a person and renders him or her unable to work varies greatly. However, is there a discrete condition of social phobia (also known as social anxiety disorder) or is this just one manifestation of the anxiety disorder that people suffer from which includes many other symptoms? How bad must my fear of public speaking become before it is branded 'abnormal'?

Normality is often determined by who is defining it, a person's value judgements and prejudices coming into play. These are important to recognise, particularly in the context of working with patients from cultures other than our own. We may have unrecognised biases against certain groups of people and therefore become more likely to think of them as abnormal because they do not live in the way that we choose to live. In the field of mental health, clinicians are more susceptible to misdiagnosis through value judgements because there is no objective test of normality but rather a sequence of symptoms and signs, perhaps backed up by health questionnaires, which lead to labelling. Throughout history, malevolent governments have declared those who do not fit in with their plans to be mentally unwell. Similarly, societies may label those who are 'socially difficult' as having a mental disorder.

A delusion is defined as a fixed false belief. Lay people commonly use the word to mean a belief that is false, fanciful or derived from deception. In medical terminology the meaning is more precise, with the implication that the belief is pathological: the result of an illness or disease process. A patient holds a delusion with absolute certainty and is not swayed by argument, however logical. However, health professionals may not always be aware of the cultural factors that should lead them to call one patient's apparent delusion a cultural norm and the same belief in another patient a sign of mental instability.

THE *DIAGNOSTIC AND STATISTICAL MANUAL OF MENTAL DISORDERS* (DSM-IV)

The DSM-IV is one of the major classification systems used in developed/ Western countries to help label patients with mental illness diagnoses. It is published by the American Psychiatric Association and uses a multidimensional or multi-axial approach to diagnosis, acknowledging that social and other factors do impact on patients' mental health (Box 9.4).[3]

To apply the diagnostic criteria to individual patients requires extensive training, according to the expert authors of the text. Health professionals have to recognise that not all patients falling into the same diagnostic category will have the same aetiology and/or precipitating factors. Moreover, they may not be suitable for the same treatment. The manual does not include advice on management. New conditions are added to the manual as considered necessary. This has led to criticism of the range of diagnoses considered to be mental disorders, as conditions are included that other clinicians are reluctant to medicalise. Examples of more controversial diagnoses include jet lag and hypoactive sexual desire disorder.

BOX 9.4 MULTI-AXIAL APPROACH TO PSYCHIATRIC DIAGNOSIS

- Axis I: Clinical syndromes
  - The clinical diagnoses, e.g. anxiety, depression, bipolar disorder.
- Axis II: Developmental disorders and personality disorders
  - Developmental disorders are those which typically become evident in childhood, such as autism and learning disabilities.
  - Personality disorders are clinical syndromes that affect a person's interaction with society. Examples are borderline personality disorder, antisocial personality disorder.
- Axis III: Physical conditions
  - These conditions affect the development, continuance or exacerbation of disorders from axes I and II. Examples are head injury and multi-infarct dementia.
- Axis IV: Severity of psychosocial and environmental stressors
  - Life events such as bereavement, moving house, becoming unemployed etc, which affect the mental condition.

Diagnosing mental illness using the DSM implies that the health professional is going to accept that the basis of mental illness is the patient's biological make-up and it is expressed in recognisable patterns of symptoms and signs. This is certainly the Western model of mental illness, and for most Western-trained health professionals it is a useful framework from which to develop a management plan. However, in many cultures a diagnosis and management plan might best begin at Axis IV rather than Axis I. So, for instance, an Aboriginal patient may have Axis IV risks of an overcrowded house, unemployment, marginalisation in the community and limited access to good food. Axis III problems may be diabetes, cataracts and deafness. Axis II disorders may stem from being part of the Stolen Generation and sexually abused as a child. Any management plan of an Axis I disorder such as depression is unlikely to be successful if the other issues are not acknowledged and addressed, beginning with the psychosocial and environmental, then the physical, the developmental and only then the clinical. Such a management plan will involve more than just one health professional and the complexities of the issues may feel overwhelming. However, dealing only with the psychiatric diagnosis denies the true nature of the patient's psychological health and well-being and is doomed to failure. Acknowledgement of the complexity of the situation and an attempt at remedying the other issues at the outset is more likely to bring some relief to the patient's distress.

There has been much criticism of the cultural inappropriateness of the DSM.[4,5] The latest version of the DSM has taken the cultural factors that might impinge on patients' mental health into account. The importance of culture is now highlighted in the introduction, the diagnostic categories and the multi-axial approach, as well as by adding a glossary of culture-related syndromes. The syndromes included in this section are not listed in the main text because the compilers feel that such conditions only occur in certain locations or within certain groups of people rather than being universal. The syndromes are also referred to as folk diagnostic categories; a label which some commentators believe implies that they have a lower status than professional labels of distress.[6] To use this glossary in an effective and ethical way, clinicians are encouraged to explore their own ethnocentric attitudes and biases. There is a recommendation to take into account not only the personal, but also the cultural perspectives of patients. However, while it incorporates cross-cultural variations in symptomatology and lists difference in prevalence rates, it ignores the possibility that standard diagnostic criteria might not be universal. It still has shortfalls, in particular in relation to the interaction of gender and culture. There is also a tendency to neglect intracultural heterogeneity.[7]

The DSM-IV does offer an extra dimension to the definition of delusion by stating that the false belief is one not ordinarily accepted by other members of the person's culture or subculture, and thus it is not an article of religious faith.

In summary, the fundamental assumptions of the DSM-IV are shown in Box 9.5.[7]

BOX 9.5 ASSUMPTIONS OF DSM-IV

- Individualist sense of self – a person should wish to be autonomous.
- Psychopathology resides in the self – rather than in interactions with external agencies.
- Disorders can be diagnosed in discrete categories.

CULTURE-BOUND SYNDROMES

The description of culture-bound syndromes implies that different cultures will have a distinctive presentation of mental illness that is peculiar to that culture, quite the opposite to the quest for screening tools whose aim is to universally pick up mental illness in all cultures. Kenneth Pike (1912–2000), a linguist and anthropologist, defined the words 'emic' and 'etic' in 1954, deriving them from phonemic and phonetic and relating them to language and linguistics (Box 9.6). He suggested that there are two perspectives that can be taken when studying a society's cultural use of language in the same way that there are two perspectives relating to a language's sound system.[8] Pike said that the native speakers of a language are the sole judges of the validity of an emic description.

BOX 9.6 EMIC AND ETIC

- **ETIC** is a general classification, objective or external view. It sees culture as a mask that is concealing universals such as psychopathology.
- **EMIC** refers to subjective understanding. It describes culture-specific psychopathology and sees culture as a fundamental source of human variation.

Screening tools search for an etic answer, culture-bound syndromes an emic answer to mental health across cultures. It is probable that neither holds the true answer but that neither is completely wrong. Culture-bound illnesses are seen as a problem in cross-cultural mental health but Marsella describes the other side of the coin when he says that 'Every time a culture disappears, the world loses an alternative way of perceiving reality and for living.'[9]

Many authorities have grappled with how culture-bound syndromes fit into the field of Western psychiatric thinking. Authorities such as Marsella[10] and Kirmayer,[11] as well as the DSM-IV,[3] outline lists and explanations of culture-bound syndromes that will not be replicated here. They discuss the symptom patterns, the causal explanations, the biological origins and the cultural overtones and ask the essentially unanswerable questions about whether there are universal psychiatric disorders that underlie all of these syndromes. There are well-recognised physiological reasons for many of the symptoms that would fit into the depression and anxiety categories of Western medicine. However, this is unlikely to help with identification or management unless therapists are aware of the culture-specific ways of expressing distress and explaining symptomatology.

Many culture-bound syndromes are based on a common aetiology rather than a pattern of symptoms. Western medicine will attribute illness to 'natural' causes such as infection, stress, organic deterioration, accident or wilful injury. Non-Western theories of 'natural' causation will include imbalance (e.g. yin and yang), nerve weakness, loss or blocking of vital energies, loss of vital essences (e.g. semen loss) or being 'hit' or 'caught' by wind. However, non-Western societies will also have supernatural theories about the cause of illness, especially mental illness. This will include mystical causations such as fate, powerful dreams, contagion from a polluting substance (e.g. menstruating woman) or mystical retribution (e.g. violation of a taboo). Other supernatural causations would be animistic (e.g. soul loss or spirit aggression) or magical causations such as sorcery, witchcraft or the 'evil eye'.[6]

The boundaries that separate sickness and health, good and bad, living and dead, natural and supernatural, seen and unseen, conscious and unconscious, dreams and reality and what is past, present and future will be different in every culture.[12] Many culture-bound syndromes or confusion about patients' diagnoses according to Western psychiatry will be because of differences in what is seen as normal and abnormal. For instance, schizophrenia is diagnosed more often in patients from cultures where hearing and seeing dead relatives is quite a common phenomenon. If the patient is also distressed about the death or is grieving, it may be very difficult to differentiate a Western diagnosis from normal cultural behaviour.

There are many illnesses, such as schizophrenia, depression and anxiety, that have been around for thousands of years. The ways they are expressed in different cultures and the aetiologies ascribed to them have differed across time and societies. There are other illnesses that seem to have disappeared or have newly appeared in DSM and the ICD (*International Statistical Classification of Diseases and Related Health Problems*).[13] These illnesses too seem to be bound by the time, politics and culture from which the classification manuals have been written. Western medicine, too, has many of its own culture-bound syndromes.

Post-traumatic stress disorder (PTSD), for instance, is one of the newer additions to DSM, having only been added to DSM-III in 1980. An 'extreme traumatic stressor' has been interpreted by some individuals and societies as being quite commonplace events such as childbirth, and the 'victim' can pursue compensation or a high moral ground on the basis of the diagnosis.[14] At the other end of the scale, it is not unexpected that those who have been traumatised or tortured by war, the truly 'extreme traumatic stressors', have a syndrome of re-experiencing the event, avoiding traumatic stimuli and physiological and psychological symptoms. To diagnose these people with an illness may be seen as explaining away the horror and misery they have experienced to a politically or medically expedient 'culture-bound' category.

The DSM-IV separates somatoform disorders and culture-bound syndromes from the more 'worthy' psychological disorders that make up the bulk of the manual. The implication is that mind and body are discrete entities and that cultures that have syndromes that combine physical and psychological symptoms are unusual. It is generally recognised, however, that somatic symptoms are an integral part of psychological distress. The basis of many forms of treatment is to interrupt the vicious cycle of social processes, 'emotional arousal, bodily focussed attention, symptom attribution, and cognitive appraisal' that can escalate the physical and psychological symptomatology.[15]

There is a growing body of neuropsychiatric and neuroevolutionary literature that struggles at a different level with the similarities and differences in the manifestation of mental illness in different cultures. Bracha discusses the evolution of psychiatric illnesses and relates them back to the development of 'harm-avoidance-related' and 'fitness-enhancing' genes in different phases in the evolution of humans.[16] He suggests that the DSM-V should classify mental illness according to neuropsychiatric and neuroevolutionary aetiologies rather than syndrome descriptions. When looking at the evolution of culture-bound syndromes, 'geographical ancestry' would best describe how the genetic component of these illnesses has developed in different areas. Specific harm-avoidance and fitness-enhancing genes will be selected out, not just because of the cultural environment, but also because of the geographical and historical situation.[16] 'Overconsolidation disorders' (e.g. PTSD, fear of dogs, fear of hospitals) are those that have been 'learned', as compared to those that are embedded in the genetic make-up (e.g. fear of heights, fear of snakes, compulsive disorders such as lock checking and hoarding and many pseudo-somatic symptoms).

However, most of these inherited behaviour traits have now outlived their usefulness and need to be treated if they are disrupting a patient's modern-day life.[16] Genetic make-up is obviously only one part of the development of psychological disposition. Early environment, social factors, the load of physical and psychological stressors, and of course culture all contribute and cannot be discounted. These factors will not only over-ride the genetic make-up, but the whole picture can be 'unlearned' with the passage of time and events or with more purposeful modification such as psychotherapy.

A therapist's main task is not to pigeon-hole the patient's illness into a clever box, but to listen to their account of their suffering, how their illness relates to their ability to function, how their culture interprets these symptoms and their society's way of dealing with it (*see* Cultural Awareness Tool, Chapter 2). It is important that the therapist doesn't somatise or medicalise an illness into a narrow framework when it has a wider social, cultural or spiritual meaning for the patient. Introducing psychological language into what is presented as a somatic illness or culture-bound syndrome may conflict with the patient's cultural understanding and cause confusion rather than healing.[15]

BOX 9.7 CASE STUDY 2

A 14-year-old boy was brought into the Emergency Department in Nepal by five elder men from a village two days' walk from the hospital. He was said to have suddenly fallen to the ground and since that moment had been mute and paralysed. He underwent many investigations in the hospital for epilepsy, brain tumour, encephalitis, infections etc but nothing was found. He gradually began to talk but did not relate normally and said he was 'numb all over' with 'jham jham' (tingling). The psychiatrist in the hospital could not find an explanation for his symptoms except to describe him as 'hysterical'.

The Australian consultant emergency doctor reviewed the patient, as he had spent two days in Emergency and needed to be discharged but was obviously still unwell. She thought it unusual for a young boy to be brought to the hospital by five senior men and asked what else had happened at the time he first became mute and paralysed. They explained that apparently a witch had jumped in front of the boy on the way to school and put a curse on him because he was being noisy outside her house. If the boy survived this curse he would be seen as someone with supernatural powers of his own.

Something had to be done. The consultant walked up to the boy, put her hand on his forehead and told him he was now well and should go back to the village and apologise to the witch. The boy immediately got out of bed and left the hospital with the five men. They thanked her and went on their way as though this was the expected outcome. The elder men behaved like this was a 'medical' problem by bringing the boy to hospital but the hospital mostly behaved like this was not a 'real illness', as it did not fit into any diagnostic category. The doctor was left asking herself all sorts of questions. Was this a culture-bound illness? Was this a hysterical conversion reaction? Was it truly a curse? Was this anxiety disorder? Was this just a very frightened boy? Did she do 'psychotherapy' on this patient or did she dispel the curse?

THE INTERNATIONAL GUIDELINES FOR DIAGNOSTIC ASSESSMENT (IGDA)

The development of these guidelines has been a collaborative project between the World Psychiatric Association (WPA) and the World Health Organization (WHO). Their purpose is an 'effective integration of universalism (which facilitates professional communication across centres and continents) and local realities and needs (which address the uniqueness of the patients in his or her particular context).'[17]

This intention mirrors the patient-centred approach advocated within primary care settings, acknowledging that the mentally ill patient is a whole person and not just a receptacle for disease. Figure 9.1 illustrates the historical, cultural and clinical bases for diagnosis and management using the IGDA guidelines.[18]

This is of course good practice; the problem is that the interviewing clinician may have no previous knowledge of this patient's cultural background or beliefs and may find it difficult to tease out the 'normal' from the possible psychiatric symptoms. Involving family and carers may make the task no easier; a patient advocate may be more helpful.

There are three main approaches to the cultural translation described, which are summarised in Box 9.8.[19]

BOX 9.8 CULTURAL TRANSLATION

- **Epidemiological and biomedical:** the condition is the same regardless of the sociocultural context.
- **Ethnographic:** studies the symptoms of the conditions in each society within its own belief and meaning systems.
- **Social constructionist perspective:** examines the conditions in the light of the society's attitudes to gender, race, class and ethnicity.

The biomedical model as outlined above derives from the scientific evidence relating to brain biochemistry and thus postulates that all human beings will have the same biological derangements underlying similar conditions. They will therefore respond on the whole to the same treatments i.e. those pharmaceutical agents developed within a biomedical framework. This is also an etic perspective. However, there is some recognition that a person's ideas and concerns about the problem may vary.

Anthropologists work on the assumptions of the ethnographic approach, adopting an emic perspective and studying each society and the symptoms of illness based on the local belief and meaning systems. Therefore, they doubt that illness can be treated by drugs developed within a different belief system and acknowledge that illness may be managed with local healing practices.

In the third approach, similarities between cultures are explored rather than differences. Thus a person from a low socioeconomic background is likely to have more in common with a similar person in another country than with a rich citizen of his own society. Similarly, gender politics and the attitudes to other minority groups such as gay and lesbian are recognised.

Kleinman coined the term 'category fallacy' in 1988 for the tendency to apply the diagnostic labels of one culture to another.[20] In these circumstances such labels may lack coherence and have no pathological basis. Thus, for example, the attempt to diagnose indigenous Australians as suffering from illnesses formulated by white Anglo-Saxon colonisers is a category fallacy.

THE HEALING ART

In 1973 the American psychiatrist Jerome Frank suggested that systems of healing in every culture share certain characteristics (Box 9.9),[21] to which we may add definitions of normal and abnormal behaviour. It is usually easier for

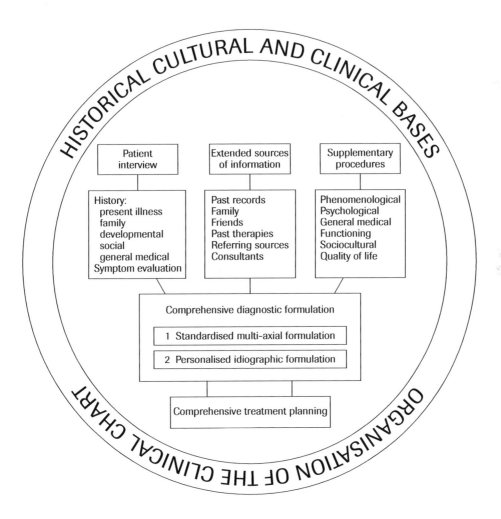

FIGURE 9.1 Approaches to the cultural translation of mental health problems[18]

a society to define illness and disease than to define what is meant by healthy, the latter often being recognised in relation to the former: health is the absence of illness. Illness represents a movement from wellness to sickness, while healing is transformation in the opposite direction. We cannot understand a patient's health beliefs without exploring both directions. The beliefs which seek to understand the change from health to illness are the foundation of what the healer must do to affect the reverse.

BOX 9.9 CHARACTERISTICS OF SYSTEMS OF HEALING

- A theory of affliction.
- Defined roles for patient and healer.
- Defined place and time for healing rituals.
- Symbolic actions with healing efficacy.
- Expectations of recovery.
- Definition of normal and abnormal/deviant.

Within the context of the 'healing art', psychotherapy may be thought of as being characterised by a healing agent (the psychotherapist is trained and sanctioned by society to act in this role), a sufferer who seeks help and a healing relationship (for example, a series of consultations between the healer and the sufferer whose aim is to bring about relief of symptoms).[22]

In a review of healing practices around the world, Kirmayer of the Division of Social and Transcultural Psychiatry in Montreal writes of the metaphors for healing and states that 'at the heart of any healing practice are metaphorical transformations of the quality of experience (from afflicted to healed) and the identity of the person (from afflicted to healed).'[22] We would also add the reverse, as people move from being considered healthy to being considered sick. A person may decide that he or she is ill but without the agreement of society, and in particular doctors, this may not be accepted. Medical certification of illness is an important role of doctors and they have the power to decide whether illness is real or illusory, though this does not rule out psychosomatic causes leading to physical disease that is diagnosed medically as due to mental illness.

For patients from different cultures this is important as their cultural norms may define health and illness from different perspectives than the society in which they are now living. To be judged as being ill in their new environment they may have to submit to the healing processes of that environment rather than their own traditional methods of healing. Often people in fact will seek help from healers in two or more different systems, and often they do not convey this state of affairs to either side.

Listening to patients' stories of their health and illness experiences is important to make sense of the metaphors and language they use to describe their state of mind and body. Understanding what this person believes is normal helps the health professional to diagnose and subsequently manage the condition that the person distinguishes as abnormal. However, the language and metaphors that patients from different cultures use may not be so easy to understand, even if there is a common verbal language.

There is also a danger of too much psychoanalysis of a person's problem. Relating a mental health problem to childhood separation from a parent, for example, may equate with one's own psychological belief systems but may be assuming too much – even with current knowledge about the limbic system. Trying to make sense of a person's symptoms following a full exploration of their life from preconception may not be helpful in management. One's own value judgements colour diagnoses of people from familiar cultural backgrounds and this may adversely affect the clinician–patient relationship. Attempting to analyse a patient from a very different culture or group is even more likely to fail.

PRACTICAL TIPS

➤ It is not always of practical or theoretical help to try to split mind and body, psychological problems and physical problems.
➤ Humans need to lay down neural pathways for healthy relationships early in life and this is helped by a nurturing environment.
➤ Sharing of information and cultural health beliefs is important in consultations.
➤ There is no one definition of normality, and certain mental health diagnoses are controversial, particularly in cultural terms.

REFERENCES

1 Whiting PW, Clouston A, Kerlin P. Black cohosh and other herbal remedies associated with acute hepatitis. *Med J Aust.* 2002; **177**: 440–3.
2 Lewis T, Amini F, Lannon R. *A General Theory of Love.* New York: Vintage Books; 2001.
3 American Psychiatric Association. *Diagnostic and Statistical Manual of Mental Disorders: DSM-IV-TR.* 4th ed. Washington DC: APA; 1994.
4 Wakefield J. Disorder as harmful dysfunction: a conceptual critique of DSM-III-R's definition of mental disorder. *Psychol Rev.* 1992; **99**: 232–47.
5 Thakker J, Ward T. Culture and classification: the cross-cultural application of the DSM-IV. *Clin Psychol Rev.* 1998; **18**: 501–29.

6 Andary L, Stolk Y, Klimidis S. *Assessing Mental Health Across Cultures*. Bowen Hills: Australian Academic Press; 2003.

7 Mezzich JE, Kirmayer JL, Kleinman A, *et al.* The place of culture in DSM-IV. *J Nerv Ment Dis*. 1999; **871**: 457–64.

8 Pike K. *Language in Relation to a Unified Theory of the Structure of Human Behaviour*. The Hague: Mouton; 1954.

9 Marsella A, Yamada A. Culture and mental health: an introduction and overview of foundations, concepts, and issues. In: Cuellar I, Paniagua F, editors. *Handbook of Multicultural Mental Health*. New York: Academic Press; 2000. pp. 3–24.

10 Marsella A. Culture and psychopathology. In: Kitayama S, Cohen D, editors. *Handbook of Cultural Psychology*. New York: Guilford Publications, Inc; 2007. pp. 797–818.

11 Kirmayer L (2001). Cultural variations in the clinical presentation of depression and anxiety: implications for diagnosis and treatment. *J Clin Psychiatry*. 2001; **62**(Suppl. 13): S22–8.

12 Nyagua J, Harris A. West African refugee health in rural Australia: complex cultural factors that influence mental health. *Rural Remote Health*. 2008; **8**(884). Available at: www.rrh.org.au/publishedarticles/article_print_884.pdf

13 World Health Organization. *International Statistical Classification of Diseases and Related Health Problems (10th revision)*. Geneva: WHO; 1992.

14 Summerfield B. The invention of post-traumatic stress disorder and the social usefulness of a psychiatric category. *BMJ*. 2001; **322**: 95–8.

15 Kirmayer L, Looper K. Abnormal illness behaviour: physiological, psychological and social dimensions of coping with distress. *Curr Opin Psychiatry*. 2006; **19**: 54–60.

16 Bracha HS. Human brain evolution and the 'Neuroevolutionary Time-depth Principle': implications for the reclassification of fear-circuitry-related traits in DSM-V and for studying resilience to warzone-related posttraumatic stress disorder. *Prog Neuropsychopharmacol Biol Psychiatry*. 2006; **30**: 827–53.

17 IGDA Workgroup, WPA. IGDA. Introduction. *Br J Psychiatry*. 2003; **182**(Suppl. 45): S37–9.

18 IGDA Workgroup, WPA, IGDA. 1: Conceptual bases – historical, cultural and clinical perspectives. *Br J Psychiatry*. 2003; **182**(Suppl. 45): S40–1.

19 Falicov CJ. Culture, society and gender in depression. *J Fam Ther*. 2003; **25**: 371–87.

20 Kleinman A. *Rethinking Psychiatry: from cultural category to personal experience*. New York: Free Press; 1988.

21 Frank JD, Frank JB. *Persuasion and Healing: a comparative study of psychotherapy*. 3rd ed. Baltimore: John Hopkins University Press; 1991.

22 Kirmayer LJ. The cultural diversity of healing: meaning, metaphor and mechanism. *Brit Med Bull*. 2004; **69**: 33–48.

10

Cross-cultural pharmacotherapy

This chapter explores:
■ Issues relating to cross-cultural psychopharmacology
■ The variation in response to medication
■ Making a decision to prescribe
■ Shared decision-making
■ Adherence to the prescribing of medication
■ Alternative or traditional medicines
■ Prescribing in depression
■ Benzodiazepines

(Note that in discussing drug treatments, we refer to the Western, conventional medicines as 'orthodox' and non-Western traditional medicines as complementary or alternative. This is fairly common usage and is not meant to be taken as a value judgement about the various systems.)

Drug treatment is a common management strategy for mental health problems. In the transcultural context the prescriber (who will usually be the doctor) needs to take into account the cultural nuances of drug taking, the differing responses of certain sections of the population to medicines (including variations between men and women) and the concerns of patients regarding medication. With regards to specific drug treatments, this chapter focuses on the commonly prescribed psychotropics: antidepressants and anxiolytics.

PHARMACOTHERAPY ACROSS THE WORLD

Western medicine has built an evidence base for the efficacy of psychotropic medication across a range of mental health problems. Most Western countries encourage and often subsidise or fund the use of these medications, ensuring that their populations have adequate mental healthcare. About 33% of countries allocate less than 1% of their total health budgets to mental health,[1] and 50% of the Western Pacific countries, most African countries and four out of nine Arab countries have no national mental health policies or programs.[2] In many developing countries there is a lack of research on mental health epidemiology, services, treatment, prevention and promotion, and policy. Without such research there is no rational basis to guide advocacy, planning and intervention.[3]

In its *New Understanding, New Hope* report, the World Health Organization (WHO) said:

> Despite the chronic and long-term nature of some mental disorders, with the proper treatment, people suffering from mental disorders can live productive lives and be a vital part of their communities. Over 80% of people with schizophrenia can be free of relapses at the end of one year of treatment with antipsychotic drugs combined with family intervention. Up to 60% of people with depression can recover with a proper combination of antidepressant drugs and psychotherapy.[3]

In most studies, only about 60% of depressed patients are recognised as having a mental health problem by their GP and only about 25% are given a specific diagnosis of depression. Less than half of those with depression are prescribed an antidepressant.[4] Up to 50% of serious cases in developed countries and 80% in developing countries receive no treatment.[5] Despite the fact that selective serotonin reuptake inhibitors (SSRIs) have been available in most countries for over a decade, tricyclic antidepressants are frequently used in low doses that are unlikely to be of benefit. In the WHO Psychological Problems in General Health Care study none of the patients in China, 1% of those in Nigeria, 5% in Chile, 8% in Brazil and 22% in Bangalore were even prescribed tricyclic medication.[6] Benzodiazepine use is particularly common in developing countries where doctors are extremely short of time and there is limited mental health training. Common reasons for not prescribing antidepressants include cost, inadequate supply, absence from the country's essential drug list, lack of training, traditional beliefs and lack of belief that antidepressants are an appropriate treatment.[2]

CROSS-CULTURAL PSYCHOPHARMACOLOGY

Cross-cultural psychopharmacology, also termed ethnopharmacology, is the study of variation between ethnic groups in relation to the efficacy of psychotropic medication. Response may be affected by psychosocial and environmental factors and, increasingly, we are becoming aware of genetic and biological factors as well, through research in the field of pharmacogenetics and pharmacokinetics. Pharmacokinetics involves the absorption, distribution, metabolism and excretion of drugs. It is the drug-metabolising enzymes under genetic control that are the most important factors in the individual and ethnic variations in drug response.[7] An obvious example of these differences is the flushing response of Asians to alcohol, caused by a genetic lack of aldehyde dehydrogenase, sometimes also coupled with an excess of alcohol dehydrogenase.[8] The discovery of genetic differences in cytochrome P-450 (CYP) enzyme systems has given scientists one explanation for variable drug dosage response. This system is responsible for the metabolism of the majority of psychotropic medications.[9] Some people may be classified as poor metabolisers and some as extensive metabolisers depending on the level of these enzymes. There is a wide range of ethnic differences in the numbers of poor metabolisers within populations.[9] Another example of such differences is slower metabolism of codeine within the Asian community potentially leading to an increased sensitivity to this commonly used drug.[9] The fact that beta-blockers are fairly ineffective in treating hypertension in African-American people is a more well-known example of this type of phenomenon.[10]

There is, however, conflicting evidence about certain drug dose responses in different ethnic groups (Box 10.1 summarises some of this evidence). A recent British paper dispelled some of the myths that Asians, Africans and Caucasians require different doses solely because of their genetic make-up. This research showed that the optimum dosage of two of the newer antipsychotic drugs (olanzapine and clozapine) is similar for all groups.[11] However, an earlier study found that about one third of African Americans are slower than the white population in metabolising psychotropic medication.[12] Too much of these drugs may therefore lead to a higher incidence of extrapyramidal side effects. The older drugs do seem to have different effects.

BOX 10.1 ETHNIC VARIATION IN DRUG METABOLISM[13]

Drug class	Effects
Benzodiazepines	Asians metabolise these slower than Caucasians
Tricyclic antidepressants	Results inconclusive
	African-Americans may be more susceptible to CNS side effects

Neuroleptics	Asians metabolise haloperidol slower than Caucasians but marked variation between individuals in both groups
Lithium	Greater toxicity noted in African-Americans Chinese patients require lower doses of lithium

There is of course a multitude of other reasons why drugs may have unpredictable effects, a variability that can be 40-fold or more (Box 10.2).[13]

BOX 10.2 FACTORS AFFECTING RESPONSE
TO PRESCRIBED MEDICATION

- Age.
- Body weight and fat ratio.
- Diet.
- Religious beliefs (e.g. fasting).
- Use of other medicines.
- Adherence to medication prescriptions.
- Placebo effect.
- Doctor's diagnosis being incorrect.
- Attitude to drug taking.
- Expectations of treatment.
- Cost and availability of medicine.

We must remember that, similar to aetiologies of mental health problems, the psychotropic drugs that are prescribed and controlled by prescribers have been developed and researched predominantly in Western cultures using 'young white male subjects'.[8] Fernando calls this imposition of alien treatment 'the imperialism of psychiatry' (p. 131).[14]

PRESCRIBING AND THE DIAGNOSIS

Doctors need to be aware of reverse labelling – a patient is diagnosed as having depression because a decision has been made to prescribe antidepressants. In fact, the underlying condition may be unhappiness related to psychosocial factors for which counselling or other therapy will offer a greater chance of relief than psychotropic medication. Some feel that the apparent increasing prevalence of depression is linked to the availability of antidepressants.[14]

People from ethnic minority groups may be given the wrong psychological diagnosis and hence the wrong medication, leading to side effects that are subsequently thought of as symptoms of the underlying erroneous condition (this of course may occur with any patient but is more likely in transcultural consultations). The wrong diagnosis may also lead in some cases to involuntary admission to a psychiatric facility. Doctors have also reported buying time with admissions in order to work out what is going on with a patient when the transcultural nuances lead to diagnostic uncertainty.[15]

THE DECISION TO PRESCRIBE

The patient-centred approach to consultations includes shared decision-making with regard to management (Box 10.3). This is particularly important when a prescription is considered, as 'telling' patients that they need to take drugs without exploring their perspectives and expectations of treatment will lead to poor adherence with medicine taking. In fact, patients may not even have their pills dispensed. The step of both the patient and doctor being involved may need to be modified to involve family members.

BOX 10.3 CHARACTERISTICS OF SHARED DECISION-MAKING[16]

- Both the patient and the doctor are involved.
- Both parties share information.
- Both parties take steps to build a consensus about the preferred treatment.
- Doctor and patient reach an agreement on the treatment to implement.

When the doctor feels that medication would be a useful adjunct to support, counselling or psychotherapy, they should explore with the patient the rationale for treatment and the patient's ideas and concerns about drug taking. Two useful questions to ask are: what does the patient think would be an appropriate treatment for this problem (this will vary between and within cultural groups) and what was the patient expecting would happen in regards to management? These questions may also have to be explored with family members if the patient consults with a relative. The steps involved in the shared decision-making process are shown in Box 10.4. As discussed in previous chapters, this process may be unusual to certain patients who may prefer a more paternalistic style of consultation. This preference should be established and indeed fits within the first two steps.

BOX 10.4 STEPS IN SHARED DECISION-MAKING[17]

- Establish a context in which patients' views about treatment options are valued and necessary.
- Elicit patients' preferences so that appropriate treatment options are discussed.
- Transfer technical information to the patient on the treatment options, risks and probable benefits in an unbiased, clear and simple way.
- Physician participation includes helping the patient conceptualise the weighing process of risks versus benefits and ensuring that their preferences are based on fact and not misconception.
- Shared decision-making involves the physician in sharing the treatment recommendation with the patient and/or affirming the patient's treatment preference.

Many patients believe that certain drugs, such as antidepressants, are 'addictive' and difficult to come off in the future. Such drugs may also be seen as symbols of mental illness. Other patients may have come to their healthcare provider specifically for drugs in the hope of cure. The patient's health beliefs, previous experiences and knowledge of friends or family members on drugs will colour expectations of treatment. Of course the psychosocial history, including the cultural background and influences, of the patient is important.

Patients in the UK have been shown to want to know about four essential aspects of their medicine (Box 10.5),[18] and these topics are obviously also important in transcultural interactions. Patients often have difficulty asking questions because they feel intimidated and are concerned about using the doctor's time;[19] or they may not have the language needed to pose certain queries. They are also not likely to remember all the information, perhaps forgetting as much as 80% of what is discussed in the consultation.[20] Therefore, leaflets in the patient's own language are useful, as well as repetition of information and checking understanding.

BOX 10.5 ESSENTIAL INFORMATION ABOUT DRUGS[18]

- Side effects.
- What it does and what it's for.
- Dos and don'ts.
- How to take it.

An additional piece of information is what the benefit of the treatment is – this is more than what the drug does. The benefit should include why this is the best drug to take and the practical experience of taking it: you will begin to feel that things are worthwhile again; you will feel less anxious. If the patient has chosen the drug from a choice of medication discussed by the doctor, this option should be ratified by saying this is a good choice. When talking about benefits, the doctor needs to make the patient aware that certain drugs take time to work; in particular antidepressants do not have a therapeutic effect for days to weeks, depending on the class. Some patients may expect to feel better immediately.

COMPLIANCE, ADHERENCE AND CONCORDANCE

One definition of compliance is the extent to which a patient's actual history of drug taking corresponds to the prescribed regimen.[21] 'Compliance' is a term often used by doctors when talking about patients and the investigations, medication and treatment arranged for them. The implication of 'poor compliance' is that the patient is not following the doctor's 'rules' because of ignorance, stupidity or laziness. There may be little acknowledgement that the 'rules' in a consultation are culturally specific, with a hierarchy and knowledge that is foreign to those from a different background.

'Adherence' is another term that has been used to describe patient behaviour.[22] However, even this increasingly popular term carries similar connotations of obeying somebody else's rules.[23]

Over 30 years ago American doctors demonstrated that adopting a patient-centred approach to consultations, including eliciting patients' worries and expectations and giving clear, jargon-free explanations of the diagnosis and its causes, improves satisfaction and compliance.[24] However, as compliance is not a patient-centred word, the newer concept of concordance is preferred to delete the impression of paternalism and 'doctor knows best'.[25] Shared decision-making appears to improve concordance and should eventually lead to a reduction in the number of unwanted drugs.[26] 'The aim of concordance is to optimise health gain from the best use of medicines, compatible with what the patient desires and is capable of achieving',[25] as well as reducing the prescription of inappropriate drugs.

PRESCRIBING ISSUES

In the treatment of mental health problems in general, women are more likely to be prescribed medication than men (and extra considerations are needed in this case – Box 10.6). Add to this the fact that patients from minority cultural backgrounds also receive more drugs, for example, in the USA, African-American patients are more likely to be treated with neuroleptics regardless of diagnosis,[27] and we can understand that the decision to recommend drug treatment is not solely based on medical need. When the patient does not have English as a first language there is also the potential for drug interactions, as the health professional may not always be aware of other medication the patient is taking – anything from other prescribed drugs, to over-the-counter medicines, to traditional medicines.

BOX 10.6 CONSIDERATIONS WHEN PRESCRIBING FOR WOMEN

- Effects on fertility.
- Interaction with contraception.
- Interaction with hormone replacement.
- Effects on menstruation.
- Possibility of pregnancy and therefore possible teratogenesis.
- Effects on libido and sexual function.
- Possible changes in weight – gain or loss.
- Effects on breast feeding.

Patients should be asked to bring any tablets, creams or potions they are using to the consultation before a prescription is given. However, sorting through these may not be easy. If drugs are not labelled or the instructions/names are in a foreign language, the ingredients may not be obvious. A pharmacist may be able to help. Ingredients and generic names of medication can often be found by searching on the internet.

THE EFFICACY OF PSYCHOTROPIC DRUGS

Drugs prescribed for mental health problems invoke emotional reactions in many people. Doctors have been accused of both over prescribing and under prescribing. There is conflict as to the extent to which drugs work compared to psychotherapeutic approaches. There may be a high degree of placebo effect involved in the response of patients. In terms of placebos, some large-scale drug trials (but over 25 years ago) have suggested that non-Caucasians may be more responsive to placebo treatment than Caucasians.[28] These sorts of results need to be treated with extreme caution and we feel should not be extrapolated to affect day-to-day practical prescribing. As might be expected the efficacy and reported incidence of side effects are heavily influenced by patients' culturally determined beliefs and expectations.[29]

ALTERNATIVE DRUG REGIMENS

In the West there is a growing awareness and seeking out of what are often now called complementary medicines. This term again reflects the orthodoxy of Western medicines, as the alternative treatments are seen as 'complementary' to the Western ones. However, in many cases they are truly alternative. Meditation and yoga, while not drugs, have been recognised as having beneficial effects on mood. The drugs of other medical and traditional systems of healing include herbal remedies, such as are used extensively in Chinese traditional medicine and the Ayurvedic system originating in India. Homeopathy, while considered alternative, was developed in the West.

In Chinese traditional medicine the physician does not prescribe for individual conditions, symptoms or signs. Rather the aim of treatment is to correct imbalance in body processes and restore harmony to the whole person. Herbs are blended for individual patients. Ayurvedic medicine also targets the individual and takes into account the patient's disposition as well as the possible illness. Herbs may be taken as pills but they may also be delivered as creams, inhalants or pessaries. The practice in the West of buying off-the-shelf herbal remedies loses sight of the fact that the prescription should be individualised. A doctor treating a patient who is also taking a traditional medicine may not be able to tell the exact ingredients within it.

Of course, as with mass-manufactured, evidence-based pharmaceuticals, there is a possible placebo effect with alternative therapies. The interaction with the healer, the words spoken, the listening process and even the laying on of hands all affect the power of the pill to restore health. This occurs in every medical arena and can be harnessed to great effect.

Patients may wish to combine a traditional healing practice or medicine with the more orthodox treatment. It is much better that the patient and doctor agree on this course of action so that the doctor is aware of what is going on rather than the two systems being used without bilateral knowledge. The transcultural prescriber needs to have an open and inquiring mind about other treatments.

PRESCRIBING IN DEPRESSION

The prescribing of antidepressant medication has become a highly political issue. At times when non-pharmacological treatments are relatively expensive and also time-consuming compared to drugs, antidepressants have not had much in the way of competition. In the United Kingdom where there is a fixed prescription charge regardless of the cost of the prescribed item, antidepressants are cheaper for the patient than their real cost. While the services of psychologists and counsellors working within the NHS are free at the point of the consultation, there is often a long wait to see them. Therefore, patients and doctors may want something that will work more quickly. In Australia, where drugs cost more on prescription, a recent government initiative has lowered the cost of psychology consultations for patients, with higher rebates available for up to 12 consultations per year, as long as a referral has been made by a GP. It remains to be seen if this has an effect on prescriptions. Moreover, not all psychologists are skilful in transcultural consultations and therefore a prescription may still seem to be a more effective form of management.

Early in 2008 a paper published in a highly regarded medical journal questioned whether there is any evidence to show that antidepressants have any major effects at all on depression, apart from in a small subset of patients with severe depression.[30] This story was picked up by the media and counter claims were made by the pharmaceutical companies, who of course make millions of pounds and dollars each year from the enormous number of antidepressants dispensed worldwide. Such media interest leads patients to question their treatment, either at the point of a management decision or after months or even years on the drugs. For patients from other cultural backgrounds who may read newspapers in their native languages, it is more difficult to know what is being written about drug treatments.

The fact that the incidence of depression and suicide in major industrial nations continues to rise has also led to questions about the efficacy of antidepressants. Drug companies have been accused of not publishing papers which show negative results in clinical trials, that is, having publication bias towards positive results. For example, one study found that only 8% of antidepressant trials with negative findings were reported as negative, while positive trials were reported 97% of the time.[31] Pharmaceutical company research has also been criticised for lack of scientific validity leading to manipulation of data, though without any specific fraudulent intent.[32] Calls have been made for independent drug research.

These debates make it more difficult to know what information to give to patients about the drug treatment of depression, particularly if they have no specific questions about it. Patients from cultures where there is rarely any challenge to a doctor's authority are less likely to seek information at the time of the consultation but they may not agree with the drug treatment option. However, when the decision is made to prescribe, within primary care settings SSRIs appear to be better tolerated than the older tricyclic group of antidepressants.[33] When considering any evidence the clinician needs to consider if the research included participants from multicultural backgrounds and thus whether it can be applied to the particular patient in the consulting room.

PRESCRIBING IN ANXIETY

Anxiolytic medication is even more controversial than antidepressants. For many years drugs such as diazepam (Valium) and nitrazepam (Mogadon) were prescribed without doctors knowing of their addictive properties. Addiction could begin within a short time of a patient starting to take them. As benzodiazepine dependence became better known, prescriptions began to be less common. While at one time benzodiazepines were the most commonly used psychotropic drugs, their ingestion has fallen steadily since the 1970s.[34] The advice now is to prescribe them for short-term control of anxiety only, for example while a patient is waiting for a psychology appointment or if symptoms are so marked as to affect day-to-day functioning, including interaction within a consultation. However, they are still very commonly prescribed in developing countries. 'The high prevalence of benzodiazepine use in primary care is especially common in developing countries. GPs state that this is partly due to the lack of time and the lack of knowledge and skills.'[35]

Anxiety is likely to be a feature of culture shock and acculturation, particularly if people have moved to a new country without complete agreement with that course of action. When prescribing any of the benzodiazepine family, patients should be warned about the sedative effects and advised about driving and operating machinery. Benzodiazepines vary in their rapidity of effect and their half-life, so the drug should be tailored to the patient's needs. They are more effective against the physical effects of anxiety such as sweating, insomnia and tremor than psychological effects such as worry and rumination. The lowest dose necessary should be prescribed and they should be used with caution in the elderly. Beta-blockers are an alternative for the physical effects if there are no contraindications for their use. SSRIs have some effects on anxiety symptoms but may take a few weeks to work.

MEDICATION FOR INSOMNIA

Before considering a drug to treat insomnia, the nature of the sleep disturbance and possible causes should be explored. 'I can't sleep' may mean very different things. Some patients complain of tiredness and a feeling that even though they sleep a lot, they wake still tired. Patients moving countries and subsequently accommodation may be unused to Western-style sleeping arrangements, may be disturbed by too much or too little noise compared to their previous homes, may have problems due to different working patterns (e.g. shifts) and/or have mental health problems affecting relaxation. Adjustment sleep disorders typically last about one week but may take longer to resolve the more complex the adjustment. Areas to explore include the onset of symptoms, whether the problem is predominantly to do with falling asleep or with waking too often (including early morning waking), whether other medication is responsible (e.g. bronchodilators, beta-blockers), whether there are nightmares and what has been tried so far. Medical reasons such as menopausal hot flushes, restless legs syndrome and sleep apnoea should be considered. Cultural factors associated with sleeping patterns should be explored, as should what the patient thinks the problem might be caused by. Anxiety and depression are common causes.

Clinicians may be able to ease the situation by discussing healthy sleeping habits (sleep hygiene) within the appropriate cultural context (Box 10.7). Suggesting that bed time should be quiet might be difficult if the patient is sharing a room with other family members.

BOX 10.7 HEALTHY SLEEPING HABITS

- Try to go to bed and get up at the same time every day.
- Avoid too much to drink before bedtime, particularly caffeine-containing drinks.
- Try not to nap during the day.
- Exercise regularly.
- Use bed only for sleeping (and sex if this is appropriate to this patient).
- Try to have exposure to bright light during the day.
- Do not go to bed too hungry or too full.
- If you do not fall asleep within 15–20 minutes of going to bed, get up and do something relaxing until you feel sleepy again.

Relaxation therapy may be helpful. Many patients ask for sleeping tablets (hypnotics); some doctors prescribe these without considering alternatives. The most commonly prescribed sleeping pills are temazepam and zolpidem. They should not be used every night and certainly not for more than two to three weeks. They should not be used with alcohol – discussing this advice needs to be done sensitively, as alcohol may be forbidden to certain groups but still might be consumed. Patients with known addiction problems should not be prescribed hypnotics. Doctors should warn about the possibility of rebound insomnia when hypnotics are stopped suddenly.

Complementary medicines are popular for the treatment of insomnia, including melatonin and valerian. Melatonin is not licensed in the UK, but it is available on prescription on a named basis, and there is little objective evidence that it works, particularly for jet lag, for which it is commonly used.

BOX 10.8 CASE STUDY 1 (NANDITA'S STORY – A PRESCRIPTION FOR ANTIDEPRESSANTS)

35-year-old Nandita was brought to the Outpatients in Nepal by her 14-year-old son, Dinesh. He was concerned that she was not looking after the house, was not eating, would get confused when she was cooking, wasn't going out at all, was up very early in the morning and was hardly speaking. He had taken her to two dhami jhankris (traditional healers) in the town and they had suggested the family make offerings in the temple. She was slowly getting worse and Dinesh had not been able to go to school, as he had to look after the house and the younger children. Indeed sitting on the stool by the desk Nandita was extremely thin and just stared blankly at the wall, her face immobile, and she was letting Dinesh do all the talking. She said she was tired all the time and was afraid her 'brain was disappearing'. Her husband was away in India working as a taxi driver and it had been two years since he had been home. As well as the children she had been caring for her mother-in-law but she had recently passed away and Nandita had become more unwell since that time.

The doctor decided that the most likely diagnosis was depression. She explained that this would feel like her 'brain was disappearing' and that there was some medication that she hoped would make it come back. Nandita was keen to try the medication and the doctor gave her an SSRI and asked her to come back in two weeks.

Nandita returned two weeks later without Dinesh. She smiled and greeted the doctor, sat down and began to describe at great length how bad she felt with back pain and stomach upset. She also talked with feeling about how disappointed she was with her husband for not coming home for his mother's funeral and with Dinesh because he kept calling her names and saying she was lazy. The doctor was quite taken aback at the dramatic change in Nandita's presentation and mentioned that she thought Nandita looked a lot better. Nandita gently chastised the doctor and said that she felt much worse than before. Then, she didn't feel anything; now, she was upset and in pain. The doctor explained that this meant that her brain was beginning to work again. Nandita looked wide-eyed at the doctor and suddenly laughed. The two could then start to talk about how so many things had piled up in Nandita's life and find ways through her current problems.

PRACTICAL TIPS

➤ Drugs have a role in the management of mental health problems but should only be prescribed after full discussion with patients.

➤ The clinician should explore the use of alternative and traditional medicines both for efficacy and in the case of drug interactions.

➤ There is some evidence that there are ethnic variations in the way that drugs are metabolised, with implications for dosage.

REFERENCES

1 World Health Organization. *Mental Disorders Affect One in Four People.* 2001 Available at: www.who.int/whr/2001/media_centre/press_release/en/ (accessed April 2008).

2 Abas M, Baingana F, Broadhead J, *et al.* Common mental disorders and primary health care: current practice in low-income countries. *Harv Rev Psychiatry.* 2003; **11**: 166–73.

3 World Health Organization. *The World Health Report 2001. Mental Health: new understanding, new hope.* Available at: www.who.int/whr/2001/en/whr01_en.pdf (accessed April 2008).

4 Lecrubier Y. Widespread underrecognition and undertreatment of anxiety and mood disorders: results from 3 European studies. *J Clin Psychiatry.* 2007; **68**(Suppl. 2): S36–41.

5 The WHO World Mental Health Survey Consortium. Prevalence, severity, and unmet need for treatment of mental disorders in the World Health Organization World Mental Health Surveys. *J Am Med Assoc.* 2004; **291**: 2581–90.

6 Ustun T, Sartorius N, editors. *Mental Illness in General Health Care: an international study.* Chichester, England: John Wiley & Sons; 1995.

7 Minas H, Silove D. Transcultural and refugee psychiatry. In: Bloch S, Singh B, editors. *Foundations of Clinical Psychiatry.* Melbourne, Australia: Melbourne University Press; 2001. pp. 475–90.

8 Rey JA. The interface of multiculturalism and psychopharmacology. *J Pharm Pract.* 2006; **19**: 379–85.

9 Pi EH, Simpson GM. Cross-cultural psychopharmacology: a current clinical perspective. *Psychiatr Serv.* 2005; **56**: 31–3.

10 Moser M, Lunn J. Comparative effects of pindolol and hydrochlorothiazide in black hypertensive patients. *Angiology.* 1981; **32**: 561–6.

11 Taylor DM. Prescribing of clozapine and olanzapine: dosage, polypharmacy and patient ethnicity. *Psychiatr Bull.* 2004; **28**: 241–3.

12 Lin KM, Poland RE, Wan Y, *et al.* The evolving science of pharmacogenetics. *Psychopharmacol Bull.* 1996; **32**: 205–17.

13 Lin KM, Poland RE. *Ethnicity, Culture and Psychopharmacology*. Available at: www.acnp. org/g4/GN401000184/CH180.html (accessed March 2008).

14 Fernando S. *Mental Health, Race and Culture*. 2nd ed. Basingstoke: Palgrave; 2002.

15 Andary L, Stolk Y, Klimidis S. *Assessing Mental Health Across Cultures*. Bowen Hills: Australian Academic Press; 2003.

16 Charles C, Gafni A, Whelan T. Shared decision-making in the medical encounter: what does it mean? (or it takes two to tango). *Soc Sci Med*. 1997; **44**: 681–92.

17 Towle A, Godolphin W, Richardson A. *Competencies for Informed Shared Decision-Making (ISDM): report on interviews with physicians, patients and patient educators and focus group meetings with patients*. Vancouver: University of British Columbia; 1997.

18 Dickinson D, Raynor DKT. Ask the patients – they may want to know more than you think. *BMJ*. 2003; **327**: 861.

19 Towle A, Godolphin W, Manklow J, *et al*. Patient perceptions that limit a community-based intervention to promote participation. *Patient Educ Couns*. 2003; **50**: 231–3.

20 Kessels RPC. Patients' memory for medical information. *J R Soc Med*. 2003; **96**: 219–22.

21 Urquhart J. Patient non-compliance with drug regimens: measurement, clinical correlates, economic impact. *Eur Heart J*. 1996; **17**(Suppl. A): S8–15.

22 Vermeire E, Hearnshaw H, Van Royen P, *et al*. Patient adherence to treatment: three decades of research. A comprehensive review. *J Clin Pharm Ther*. 2001; **26**: 331–42.

23 Benson J. Concordance – an alternative to compliance in the Aboriginal population. *Aust Fam Physician*. 2005; **34**: 831–4.

24 Korsch BM, Gozzi EK, Francis V. Gaps in doctor–patient communication. *Pediatrics*. 1968; **42**: 855–71.

25 Marinker M. Personal paper: writing prescriptions is easy. *BMJ*. 1997; **314**: 747–8.

26 Royal Pharmaceutical Society of Great Britain. *From Compliance to Concordance: achieving shared goals in medicine taking*. London: RPSGB; 1997.

27 Mendoza R, Smith MW, Poland RE, *et al*. Ethnic psychopharmacology: the Hispanic and Native American perspective. *Psychopharmacol Bull*. 1991; **27**: 449–61.

28 Escober JI, Tuason VB. Antidepressant agents: a cross cultural study. *Psychopharmacol Bull*. 1980; **16**: 49–52.

29 Lin KM, Poland RE, Nakasaki G. *Psychopharmacology and Psychobiology of Ethnicity*. Washington DC: American Psychiatric Press; 1993.

30 Kirsch I, Deacon BJ, Huedo-Medina TB, *et al*. Initial severity and antidepressant benefits: a meta-analysis of data submitted to the Food and Drug Administration. *PLoS Med*. 2008; **5**(2): e45

31 Turner EH, Matthews AM, Linardatos E, *et al*. Selective publication of antidepressant trials and its influence on apparent efficacy. *N Engl J Med*. 2008; **358**: 252–60.

32 Procopio M. The multiple outcomes bias in antidepressants research. *Med Hypotheses*. 2005; **65**: 395–9.

33 MacGillivray S, Arroll B, Hatcher S, *et al*. Efficacy and tolerability of selective serotonin reuptake inhibitors compared with tricyclic antidepressants in depression treated in primary care: systematic review and meta-analysis. *BMJ*. 2003; **326**: 1014–17.

34 Tiller JW. Reducing the use of benzodiazepines in general practice. *BMJ*. 1994; **309**: 3–4.

35 Lotrakul M, Saipanish R. *Psychiatr Serv in Primary Care Settings: a survey of general practitioners in Thailand*. 2006. Available at: www.biomedcentral.com/1471-2296/7/48 (accessed April 2008).

11

Cross-cultural learning

This chapter explores:
- The importance of cross-cultural learning
- Definitions
- Cultural competency
- Exploring health beliefs in a culturally sensitive way
- Cultural and racial barriers in the consultation
- Race equality training
- Learning to work with interpreters
- More on culture shock
- Language, jargon and slang
- Experiential learning

In recognition of the multicultural societies in which Western health professionals live and work there has been an increasing interest and necessity for all health professionals to learn about the different cultures from which their patients come and/or the culture in which they are working if different from their own. This is important for any patient–professional encounter but there are additional difficulties when dealing with mental health problems. Most clinicians, unless working within a narrow speciality or field, should be able to recognise mental distress and either help the patient themselves or know to whom to refer. However, when cultural influences are factored into the consultation, such recognition becomes more difficult and may be delayed, particularly if the professional concentrates on making sense of physical symptoms by looking for a physical cause. As we have discussed in earlier chapters, the Western tradition of separating mind and body is a potent factor leading to frustration of both the professional and patient, notwithstanding the almost universal agreement as to the presentation of psychosomatic symptomatology.

One of the tenets of cross-cultural learning is that the subjective experience of illness is related to culture, including symptom recognition and help-seeking by patients.[1]

As with any other educational endeavour, new ways of using old words have emerged – cross-cultural teaching has its own jargon, as displayed in the literature. While cultural diversity courses do not necessarily concentrate on mental health problems, one of their hallmarks is the focus on a patient-centred approach, which often includes exploring a patient's narrative. Such a narrative or story will, of course, be strongly influenced by its narrator's cultural background and upbringing.

THE IMPORTANCE OF CROSS-CULTURAL LEARNING

In the developed world, health statistics highlight the disparity between the well-being of the predominantly white/European ancestral origins population of those countries (e.g. Europe, Canada, the United States, Australia) and the people often referred to as 'ethnic minorities', though this also includes the indigenous inhabitants of colonised continents. Such inequalities 'result from inextricably linked, complex factors including historical and current racism',[2] and from individuals, institutions, the media and wider society. Factors contributing to these inequalities are barriers to routine access to health promotion and disease prevention interventions through lack of awareness, low income and/or language difficulties, and the lack of cultural awareness by many health professionals. To overcome these barriers, at least partially, there has been a growing awareness of the importance of cross-cultural and race equality training/learning. Such learning is important because the ability of people to recognise symptoms of ill health and to seek help is culturally defined, as is the maintenance of good-health.[1] To improve cross-cultural interactions between patient and health professional, the clinician needs to be able to integrate the multiple cultures in the encounter: his or her own culture, that of the patient/carer/family and that of the healthcare service/institution.[3]

Cross-cultural training should help health professionals move away from the notion that the health beliefs of patients arising from their cultural background are always likely to be a hindrance, if not overtly harmful, to an understanding that such beliefs may be therapeutic. As 95% of disease stems from environment and lifestyle factors (with only 5% having a genetic aetiology), we cannot practise medicine in a multicultural society without opening our minds to the cultural nuances of our patient/client base.

All health professionals should have grounding in cross-cultural understanding. The depth of this understanding needs to take into account the clientele with whom the professional works and the type of clinical interactions undertaken. Psychotherapists working with patients from different cultural backgrounds will need more extensive knowledge and skills to manage the intricacies of mental health problems presenting to them. This applies also to therapists from other cultures and countries who come to practise in a Western society.

DEFINING CROSS-CULTURAL LEARNING AND TEACHING, AND TERMS

The term cross-cultural means combining or contrasting two or more cultural groups. However, culture itself is not always easily defined. When running cultural diversity workshops, a good opening ice-breaker is to ask the group for its understanding of culture, then to ask each individual what he or she would identify as his or her culture or cultural background. Many people will give more than one – sometimes identifying as being from a nation (e.g. English), sometimes relating to a religion (e.g. Muslim), or a mix such as British Asian etc. There may even be someone who says he is from an alternative culture such as 'travellers' in the UK.

Some definitions of terms are given in Box 11.1.

BOX 11.1 DEFINITIONS RELATING TO CULTURAL DIVERSITY

- **Culture:** The total way of life – the underlying pattern of thinking, feeling and acting – of particular groups of people.[4] How people make sense of their surroundings, including attitudes and behaviour, assumptions and values. What people 'take for granted', what they notice about others but is largely invisible to themselves. The interaction between language, social structure, religion, world view, environment, economy, technology, belief and values.[5] Culture is not the same as race or ethnicity.
- **Multiculturalism:** An ideology advocating that society should consist of, or at least allow and include, distinct cultural groups, with equal status.[6] This is not an ideology to which everyone or every state ascribes.
- **Cultural awareness:** Knowing and understanding that there is a difference between people or cultural diversity; having insight into the physical, psychological, social, spiritual, economic and political context in which people live or have lived.
- **Cultural competence:** Competence itself has been defined as the ability to assume a combination of well-defined roles.[7] Cultural competency may

therefore be defined as being able to give direct patient care to people from different cultural backgrounds. In the literature this is the term often used as a learning outcome for cultural diversity training.

- **Cultural sensitivity:** Insight into and reflection on how our own and others' culture affect our interactions and behaviour.
- **Cultural relativity:** Understanding the cultural development of societies without trying to impose absolute moral ideas or trying to compare cultures against some form of absolute cultural standard.
- **Cultural intelligence:** Engaging and balancing the head, heart and mind in new and/or uncomfortable cross-cultural situations.[8]
- **Cultural safety:** An environment that is safe for people: where there is no challenge to, assault on or denial of their identity, of who they are and what they need. There is shared respect, shared meaning, shared knowledge and shared experience in addition to learning, living and working together with dignity and true listening.[9] Health professionals should be able to provide such an environment when interacting with their patients.
- **Culturally inclusive environment:** In such an environment people from any cultural background can freely express who they are, give their own opinions and points of view; may fully participate in teaching, learning, work, social activities and healthcare, can feel safe from abuse, harassment or unfair criticism.[10]

When thinking about cultural diversity training we often assume that it is the health professional who is 'native' and the patient/client who is 'foreign' or from a different culture. However, there are two fallacies arising from this assumption. Firstly, health professionals differ widely in their cultural backgrounds whether they are from the country in which they are working or whether they are immigrants into it. Secondly, on the other hand, health professionals trained in different countries but within a biomedical, orthodox or Western model, may have very similar outlooks on patient care, at odds with those of the patients with whom they interact. In some ways health professionals also enter a culture of their own, with its code of conduct, dress standards and jargon. The underlying message here is: never assume but always explore.

CULTURAL COMPETENCY

Cultures are dynamic and are influenced by other cultures around them. While we can learn certain aspects of religious or ethnic lifestyles such as dietary taboos, funeral customs and communication rituals from books, the best way to try to understand our patients or our doctors is through direct experience. However, such experience is unlikely to be best assimilated 'on the job' without support. It is very easy to offend through ignorance and even more so when interacting with a patient who is mentally and/or physically unwell.

Learning lists of so-called cultural norms may lead to stereotyping. Indeed cultural competency training has been criticised as an attempt, while trying to ensure that medical students and doctors no longer hold ignorant or biased views about their patients, to reduce cultural issues to an overly simplistic level.[11] It is all too easy to attribute to one person the customs and attitudes of a whole group of people because of a few similarities. Education that focuses only on specific attributes and differences tends to distract students and health professionals from reflecting on their own attitudes and biases.[12]

We know from our own experiences that our friends, relatives and other acquaintances who appear to be from the same 'cultural background' as ourselves may hold very different opinions from our own. Even our health beliefs may vary – one may have complete and utter faith in their homeopathic practitioner while another sees all that falls outside of orthodox Western medical practice as 'quackery'. A study of British Bangladeshi patients with diabetes found that not only their cultural background, but also their social circumstances and socioeconomic status affected their attitudes towards their condition. Similar levels of deprivation to their non-Bangladeshi neighbours meant that the two groups shared many beliefs about diabetes. The similarities were as striking as the differences in health beliefs between the two groups.[13] Some people who migrate to another culture will quickly and easily seem to assimilate into the new culture, some will incorporate features from both cultures into a 'third' or 'hybrid' culture and some will maintain most of the features of their original culture. Cross-cultural education should therefore also address social factors such as level of education, living standards, income, religion and support networks.[14]

Health professional students and practitioners should attend cultural diversity training to discuss both generic competencies and those specific to the patient groups with whom they work. They need to recognise that diversity involves not only cultural differences, but ethical and moral ones as well. Irvine and colleagues from the University of Newcastle, New South Wales, do not believe that contemporary biomedical ethics has 'adequately engaged with indigenous and non-Western ethical frameworks and modes of moral thought'.[15] To overcome this, professionals should be able to recognise and reflect on their own potential prejudices and assumptions.

Topics for discussion at introductory cultural diversity/safety workshops are suggested in Box 11.2. These should be tailored to suit local needs and run as interactive sessions. Participants should be able to challenge each other if unhelpful or harmful statements are made. It is important to establish ground rules at the beginning of the sessions. While the ground rules ideally should be set by the participants, they should include respect for each other, confidentiality and how statements may be challenged.

BOX 11.2 IDEAS FOR DISCUSSION AT DIVERSITY WORKSHOPS

- Definitions (as above in Box 11.1).
- Discussion of one's own culture and what this means.
- How one's own culture may affect one's professional practice.
- How to be culturally aware and provide a culturally safe environment for professionals and patients.
- Communication and potential problems.
- Working with interpreters.
- Use and meaning of jargon and slang.
- Possible differences in health beliefs in cultural groups and how this might affect accessing healthcare.
- Gender differences and how this might affect professional–patient interactions.
- Family structure and dynamics and their bearing on healthcare.
- Confidentiality: does this differ?
- Treatment of children and the elderly.
- Attitudes to medicine taking and modes of delivery.

With regards to specific groups, health professionals should be aware of common beliefs, with an understanding that these should be checked, as they cannot be assumed for any individual. Knowledge of dietary restrictions, customs regarding birth and death and traditional medical practices are important. However, cultural traditions may be blurred for second and subsequent generations, for example the British-born children of Asian, African or Caribbean families may be subtly or grossly different from their parents. But professional behaviour is such that if a health worker does not know, he or she should ask in a polite way. The professional should also ensure that the patient understands what is happening and has time and opportunity to ask questions.

EXPLORING HEALTH BELIEFS IN A CULTURALLY SENSITIVE WAY

The patient-centred approach to consultations is an appropriate method of interaction when there are cultural and/or ethnic differences between patient and health professional (though in some situations a family-centred process is more appropriate). Exploring a patient's ideas, concerns and expectations is important in any consultation and this model translates well when wishing to provide culturally competent healthcare. Language may also be a barrier and an interpreter may be required (*see* Chapter 8 for more on this). However, even if language is not seen to be a problem, a patient's ideas and concerns may appear very different from those of one's own background.

Health professionals trained in the Western biomedical tradition may be used to 'old wives tales' regarding diagnosis and treatment, as they have probably been exposed to such beliefs from childhood. However, when interacting with patients from other medical traditions many of their explanations for illness and disease may seem very strange. Explanations that one has heard during clinical practice may be discussed in a learning group and the reasons why they appear strange or exotic explored. Then think of some of the medical traditions that Western orthodox practice upholds – how might these explanations appear odd to a patient? For example, in many countries there is very little screening – think of how to explain to a women the need for a cervical (pap) smear and how one is taken or how to explain that ringworm is not caused by a worm.

As good communicators we try to adopt a patient-centred approach. Ask learners to think of times when they have tried to apply the patient-centred model and explore the patient's ideas but this has not been successful because the patient is from a culture where the doctor is regarded as a figure of authority, not to be questioned. Some patients may expect a paternalistic healer and be unprepared for sharing decisions and/or choosing options. Box 11.3 lists some of the areas that should be explored by health professionals with patients, and which should also be discussed at workshops. One useful question is: 'what methods or tools can I, as your health provider, use to help you learn more about your current illness or surgery?'[16]

BOX 11.3 AREAS TO EXPLORE IN CONSULTATIONS

- What the patient identifies as his/her cultural group.
- Length of time in this country (born here, immigrated).
- Previous experiences of medical treatment in home country/host country.

- Use of 'traditional' medicines or alternative medical practices.
- Spiritual beliefs and how these may impact on illness.
- Who else is involved in making decisions about healthcare (e.g. family, priest, religious mentor)?
- The meaning of this illness to the patient.
- Health beliefs.

OUTCOMES OF CULTURALLY SENSITIVE INTERACTIONS

Kagawa-Singer and colleagues of UCLA suggest that there are four possible outcomes of patient-doctor interactions (Box 11.4), with the last being the preferred (and indeed this outcome is the best for most consultations, including those without overt cultural differences between the participants). Number four is very similar to the shared decision-making process within a patient-centred consultation.

Number four also recognises that the clinician has his or her own cultural influences and is not therefore culturally neutral. Cultural neutrality is not helpful. 'A therapist who claims cultural neutrality . . . robs the client of the opportunity to speculate or to make observations about the therapist's background, particularly if this has an effect on the therapy in terms of connection or fit.'[17] Neutrality is indeed very difficult to maintain in any case, as the therapist inadvertently may display prejudice or racism. For transcultural therapy to have a chance of being successful, the social reality of race and racism must be acknowledged.[17]

BOX 11.4 POSSIBLE OUTCOMES OF PATIENT–DOCTOR INTERACTIONS (ADAPTED FROM KAGAWA-SINGER AND KASSIM-LAKHA)[3]

---

1 The doctor works exclusively within the biomedical model.
2 The patient and doctor function exclusively within their own cultures.
3 The doctor works within the patient's cultural framework.
4 The patient and doctor negotiate between their concepts of the cause of the problem/illness/disease and the most appropriate management to reach mutually desirable goals.

CULTURAL AND RACIAL BARRIERS IN THE CONSULTATION

The expectation of paternalism may also occur in the opposite direction. Doctors trained in some countries may be used to acting as 'father figures' and consulting in a paternalistic way. They may not be used to patients questioning their management or judgement or wishing to be involved in decision-making. Patients who acquiesce to such paternalism in the consultation may then decide not to take their medicine as prescribed or not to follow the doctor's advice. This will of course happen without the doctor's awareness and ultimately there is confusion as to what is really happening with the management plan. Patients who do not like a particular doctor's style, and who have the luxury of choice of healthcare provider, may not return for follow-up. Ways of learning that help professionals consider their consultation styles include discussion of case histories – what would you do next and why, simulated consultations with taping and feedback, and taping of 'real consultations' from clinical practice (with the consent of the patient).

The patient–doctor consultation diagnostic process involves listening and facilitating the patient's narrative. Busy doctors often do not make time to listen and use their pattern-recognition clinical diagnostic skills to reach an early conclusion as to what is the matter with the patient. Such pattern recognition is more difficult if the doctor and patient, while ostensibly speaking the same language, use very different vocabulary to describe symptoms. This can lead to misunderstandings and frustration, and a doctor becomes more likely to treat symptoms rather than explore and manage underlying causes. In these circumstances it is easy to signpost the end of a consultation with a prescription, which may indeed have been the expectation of the patient. However, medicine is often only going to provide temporary relief.

It has been said that 'cultural differences and ignorance create racism, and indifference nurtures it'.[18] Racial barriers to therapy are often more difficult to acknowledge and can occur in both directions between patient and therapist. Some patients do not want to see a doctor/clinician/therapist of a different 'colour' to themselves. While health professionals may not wish to collude with such racism, if this presents a barrier to successful treatment it has to be dealt with. Cross-cultural training should help the professional to raise the subject of difference in the consultation – one such difference is race[17] (but may be gender). The psychotherapist Lennox Thomas (of the Intercultural Therapy Centre in London) writes: 'It should be our duty to ask the clients whether or not they feel comfortable and if they are worried about the issues surrounding our race or skin colour as therapists', which can work with racial differences on either side of the therapeutic relationship. However, he goes on to state that 'It is most important that therapists can give clients permission to talk about racial persecution or discrimination, since they are the people with power in the consulting room.'[17] This is of course true in the majority of cases but does not deal with the situation where the patient is from the dominant culture/race of the country and the professional/therapist is from the minority and/or is an immigrant into the country. In this case the professional may be more familiar with racial discrimination, which may occur again in this consultation.

RACE EQUALITY TRAINING

Cross-cultural training needs to address the issues of racism and prejudice. This is more challenging than acknowledging and discussing culture and tradition. Racial prejudice and racism are related concepts with subtle differences in meaning. Racial prejudice arises from attitudes and beliefs, is often based in misperception and ignorance and may be caused by insecurity.[19] Racism is an ideology and political stance, arising from assumptions about inferior and superior races, with undertones of power and domination. It may be the result of social conditioning and history.[19] Thus racial prejudice is the feeling and racism the behaviour.

Race equality training aims to promote racial equality in a productive, practical and creative way, enabling participants to tackle both personal discrimination and institutional racism.[20] 'The most important part of the training is the development of personal understanding of institutional processes that perpetuate racism, through exploration of individual feelings about issues and (more importantly) about personal professional practice.'[20] To achieve this means moving beyond a cultural approach and the view that 'knowing about' a black person's culture inevitably leads to a non-racist stance. 'The fundamental problem of a cultural approach without an understanding of the effects of racism on the lives of black people is that an erroneous assessment of their needs is very likely to result.'[20] The effects of racism on health professionals need also to be explored in such training.

It is also interesting to note that some health professionals have been found to be reluctant to ask about a patient's ethnic origin for fear of offending him or her.[21] Health professionals, and students, may need to discuss their fears of being thought of as racist, and to explore with patients in a non-threatening environment ways in which such questions may be asked and issues about culture explored sensitively and safely.

LEARNING TO WORK WITH INTERPRETERS

One learning session may involve health professionals working with simulated patients and interpreters. The discussion could include the fact that a patient who is able to supply their name, address, date of birth and other predictable information may not have adequate English skills to take part in a medical consultation. Even having social conversation skills does not always mean that the person understands complex information in spoken or written English and they may not be able to give informed consent. In times of illness, crisis or traumatic or emotionally-charged situations, English competency may decrease dramatically.[22]

When using an interpreter, health professionals should learn to speak slowly and directly to the patient, not the interpreter or the telephone. It is important to keep short the amount to be interpreted, to speak in the first person, use short sentences, a normal tone of voice, good grammar, as little jargon as possible and a vocabulary free of complex words or colloquialisms. The professional needs to be aware of their own body language and watch the patient's body language as they are listening and speaking, as they would in a usual consultation.

The correct use of interpreters will improve the health professional's understanding of the patient, the patient's communication to the health professional, the cultural safety, the legal security and the therapeutic alliance. However, they will also improve the mutual respect of patient and therapist, build a deeper relationship, allow more humour and generally decrease the differences between the two.

INTERNATIONAL MEDICAL GRADUATES (IMGs) – DIFFICULTIES WORKING WITHIN A NEW COUNTRY

Doctors and health professionals who move to another country to work have many obstacles to overcome apart from potential miscommunication with patients from different cultures. They may be battling with the bureaucratic red tape of professional registration and visas. They may have left their own country for reasons other than a potential increase in their quality of living – they may come from a politically unstable regime or be refugees from persecution. Whatever their motivation, they are likely to be suffering from some degree of culture shock. When people move to a new job, a new country and a new healthcare system, often after an initial period of anticipation and euphoria they may become unhappy or uncomfortable. Culture shock is the anxiety arising from the experience of change from familiar surroundings, customs, ways of working and patient interaction. Even the names of drugs and dosages may be different. Worrying about working practices adds to the sense of dislocation and impedes concentration on the patients' problems. However, the professionals' recognition of culture shock and its effects on performance, if handled correctly, should build empathy with patients going through similar experiences. The important phrase here is: if handled correctly. Unfortunately, culture shock is often ignored or mishandled.

Culture shock can affect a person's emotions, behaviour and physical health. Uncertainty and bewilderment usually settle within three to six months if the person adapts to the change in circumstances. Orientation of health professionals to their new workplace is important and should be mandatory: the organisation (hospital, clinic, general practice etc) should arrange sessions and make sure that their employees have time to attend. Box 11.5 shows ways in which colleagues, friends or the institution may respond and help deal with culture shock, as well as what an individual may do to help him or herself.

BOX 11.5 OVERCOMING CULTURE SHOCK – ISSUES TO DISCUSS AT ORIENTATION – FOR ORGANISERS AND PARTICIPANTS

- Be welcoming.
- Take time to get to know new people.
- Organise social events (check diet and drink prohibitions).
- Attend social events.
- Smile.
- Ensure that support mechanisms are in place and that people know how to access them.
- Keep in contact with old friends and family.
- Exercise, as this helps reduce stress.
- Give details on how to register with a local GP.
- Register with a GP.
- Hold orientation sessions for new people, including cultural diversity training relevant to the patient demographic.

THE STYLE OF MEDICAL PRACTICE

The style of medical practice for many IMGs is likely to be very different, particularly for those who come from Asia and the Middle East. The use of open-ended questions, reflective listening skills, empathy and rapport-building were the main communication difficulties identified in one study.[23] IMGs were also more concerned about violating gender and cultural barriers and were fearful of offending patients, especially those with psychosocial issues.[23] Training and development organisations should take note of the research and resources that are available to help address clinical skills, cross-cultural issues, settlement difficulties, orientation to the health system and communication differences.[24]

For many IMGs who have been highly-paid and respected professionals in their country of origin, being a general practitioner in a country town is an enormous change in lifestyle and status. Added to the social isolation from family, culture and often religion, the prospect of failing to live up to financial, personal, family and social expectations makes IMGs at high risk for anxiety and depression. This may isolate them even further and present as withdrawal, arrogance or disinterest.[23] These issues need to be discussed sensitively and empathically with the help of a skilful facilitator.

JARGON AND CULTURE-SPECIFIC LANGUAGE

A good ice-breaker at the start of a session is to give participants examples of local language, written and verbal (for differences in dialect) and to ask for possible translations. In most cultures there are specific words, phrases and metaphors that are peculiar to particular areas and subcultures. This is no different in the many English-speaking countries of the world. It is important not to assume that 'I think my ticker's on the blink' (I think there is something wrong with my heart) is an intelligible statement in a country other than Australia or that 'This sprog is peely-wally' (This baby is unwell – said during a ward round in Cambridge) means anything outside the UK. If a health professional is working in a different culture, it is important to learn as much of the local 'dialect' as possible. Similarly, it is imperative that health professionals do not use jargon or local vernacular when speaking to patients from a different culture, even if that culture has English as a first language. A mother from the UK is likely to take offence at an Australian doctor telling her that her child is 'crook' (sick) and an English-speaking doctor from India may be confused when a Canadian tells them that 'I'm so miffed because I yaked all over the old lady's chesterfield' (I'm really upset because I vomited on my mother's couch).

Interactions with simulated patients or role play are useful ways to appreciate the pitfalls of jargon – both the patient's and the health professional's. It is imperative that health professionals do not pretend that they know what patients are talking about if they are using slang. Not only should health professionals ask but they should also check back with patients what it is they have said. In certain circumstances, if the health professional is still unsure of the meaning and context of the word, phrase or metaphor, they can check with the cultural mentor. This will need to include who is allowed to use this word, in what circumstances and to whom it can be said.[25] Adolescent patients would not expect a health professional to greet them with 'Hey dude, how's it hanging?' (Hello, how are you going?) but might expect them to know what this means.

This is important when teaching, as students from other cultures are unlikely to have an immediate understanding of local slang. If there are a lot of students or IMGs in a teaching setting, then it behoves the institution to run courses or develop resources on local dialects. In many parts of Australia there are local courses run by such organisations as the General Practice Training Programmes on local slang.[25] There are also courses run for native English speakers to be able to say at least a few words in such languages as Hindi and Urdu.

There may also be customs that a teacher should learn so as to facilitate an uninterrupted and smooth learning environment. For instance, many Muslim learners will want to break at the appropriate times for prayer but the amount of time they need might be able to be negotiated. There may be taboo relationships in a group of students that means that certain people should not sit with each other, speak to each other or touch each other. If possible, these should be clarified with a cultural mentor beforehand.

When using interpreters it is also important to be aware of slang, jargon and cultural metaphors. Asking a patient if they feel like they are 'at the crossroads', 'up the creek without a paddle' or being 'driven up the wall' may not only be difficult to interpret, but may have no meaning for someone who has lived in the desert for most of their life. As well as being sure that medical jargon, slang and cultural metaphors are not being used by the health professional, the translation of slang and cultural metaphors back to the health professional can also prove difficult. Again, where possible, a direct interpretation followed by clarifying questions and checking that the meaning is clear is best. Such a process will usually generate quite a bit of humour, as most slang and metaphors are so embedded into the culture that their origins are lost and their meaning is cumbersome to explain.

EXPERIENTIAL LEARNING FOR THE DEVELOPMENT OF CULTURALLY SENSITIVE SKILLS

While theoretical knowledge of mental health issues, including presentation and management strategies, may be gained by reading books, the best way to consolidate such learning is to practise consultation skills. Here we have to be careful of our definition of 'practise'. In the educational sense this should mean learning through graded experience rather than 'practising' on distressed patients in real-life consultations. Experiential learning involves learning through action and reflection and if possible by being observed and given feedback. Health professionals in the early parts of their careers should expect to be supervised and have the opportunity for regular case review. More senior practitioners whose clinical interactions begin to involve patients from other cultures should also consider engaging in educational sessions that will approve their cultural sensitivity. This may be required if a doctor moves from a rural area with a certain population demographic to an urban area in which there is a high percentage of patients from other cultures, including refugees and migrants. Similarly, a doctor moving to work in a new country should have orientation and educational sessions to introduce him or her to the new patient mix.

Graded experiential sessions could follow the timeline shown in Box 11.6. These would build on the cultural diversity and racial equality sessions described above. These sessions are the ideal scenario but, of course, time constraints, motivation, resources, work and other commitments and organisational demands are such that the ideal is rarely provided.

BOX 11.6 EXPERIENTIAL LEARNING SESSIONS

- Setting the scene – overview of the educational activities.
- Update of theoretical knowledge.
- The experiential learning model.
- Observation of intercultural consultations (video or with simulated patients).
- Discussion and feedback.
- Consultations with simulated patients.
- Discussion and feedback.
- Work-based consultations – observed or videotaped.
- Discussion and feedback.
- Ongoing supervision or mentoring, depending on previous experience.
- Opportunity for case discussion.
- Working through difficult 'real' cases with simulated patients.

There are a number of benefits from working with simulated patients (Box 11.7). However, learners who are not familiar with this method need to have time to adjust. Doctors trained overseas may not have as much experience of this type of educational activity and may feel threatened by being observed consulting. They may also find it difficult to accept feedback from 'the patient'.

DEVELOPING PATIENT ROLES AND SCENARIOS

The simulated patient roles should be as authentic as possible, avoiding stereotyping and caricature. However, the interactions are simulated and will always have some artificiality due to location, timing, observation or breaking down encounters into smaller chunks to match particular learning outcomes.

BOX 11.7 BENEFITS OF WORKING WITH SIMULATED PATIENTS

- Facilitator and learner have some control over environment.
- Can plan specific learning outcomes by use of scenarios, unlike opportunistic consultations in real clinical settings.
- Ability to stop consultation at learning points if patient/learner distressed.
- May re-run consultation to try different strategies.
- Immediate feedback from patient.
- Feedback from group.
- Learners can practise difficult consultations without risk of upsetting real patients.
- Scenarios may be developed in response to learner's needs.

To help achieve authenticity, roles may be based on real-life patient encounters. All doctors and health professionals have a bank of patient encounters on which to draw. These are more educationally useful if the outcome of the interaction is known in the short and long-term. However, they still only give the viewpoint of the professional, and the simulated patient who is developing the role may be able to offer different insights into patient behaviour from the perspective of being a patient. Often scenarios are based on an amalgam of patients and these have to be checked carefully for authenticity. Care also needs to be taken that patients may not be identified from these roles: some aspects of the story may need to be changed.

THE PATIENT VOICE FOR DEVELOPING SCENARIOS

Groups of real patients working with simulated patients develop authentic roles based on their stories and work through the many different ways that they could unfold with different professionals. This allows real patient ideas and concerns to be discussed and written into the scenarios. People from different cultural backgrounds should be recruited as simulated patients to help develop culturally appropriate scenarios. Self-help groups may wish to be involved in discussing their experiences, their symptoms, their concerns and the impact of any treatment they have received. Patients with a history of mental health problems may be more difficult to recruit for this work but offer great insights into their experiences and their interactions with health professionals.

BOX 11.8 CASE STUDY 1 (THE PROFESSOR'S STORY – EVEN TRAINED EDUCATORS NEED CULTURAL AWARENESS)

(WITH THE KIND PERMISSION OF PROFESSOR KONRAD JAMROZIK)

The new professor was teaching a group of students in Papua New Guinea. In the interests of getting to know each other better he asked that each student stand up and say their name and say something about themselves in front of the rest of the class. There was a great deal of discomfort at this request.

Such a simple activity was actually quite culturally inappropriate in this environment as, for certain tribes in PNG, a person is not allowed to say their own name out loud. The professor only found this out later when he discussed the incident with a 'cultural mentor' in the community.

PRACTICAL POINTS

➤ Courses on cultural diversity and communication skills are often run through postgraduate education centres.
➤ Racial equality training is important and should be available to all health professionals.
➤ Transcultural learning needs to be complemented with experiential learning and feedback to enhance performance.
➤ Patient feedback is an important part of experiential learning.
➤ Frank and open discussion of feelings in a non-threatening environment is conducive to learning but requires expert facilitation.

REFERENCES

1 Angel R, Thoits P. The impact of culture on the cognitive structure of illness. *Cult Med Psychiatry.* 1987; **11**: 465–94.
2 Bhopal R. Spectre of racism in health and health care: lessons from history and the United States. *BMJ.* 1998; **316**: 1970–3.
3 Kagawa-Singer M, Kassim-Lakha S. A strategy to reduce cross-cultural miscommunication and increase the likelihood of improving health outcomes. *Acad Med.* 2003; **78**: 577–87.
4 O'Hara-Devereaux M, Johansen R. *Globalwork: bridging distance, culture and time.* San Francisco, CA: Jossey-Bass; 1994.
5 Hammond P. *An Introduction to Cultural and Social Anthropology.* New York: McMillan; 1978.

6 Wikipedia contributors. Multiculturalism. *Wikipedia, The Free Encyclopedia*. Available at: http://en.wikipedia.org/wiki/Multiculturalism (accessed July 2007).

7 Schuwirth LWT, van der Vleuten CPM. Changing education, changing assessment, changing research. *Med Educ*. 2004; **38**: 805–12.

8 Earley C, Ang S. *Cultural Intelligence: individual interactions across cultures*. California: Stanford; 2003.

9 Williams R. *Working in a Culturally Safe Environment*. 2002. Available at: www.flinders. edu.au/kokotinna/SECT04/OVERVW.htm (accessed July 2005).

10 Flinders University. *Cultural Diversity and Inclusive Practice Toolkit*. Available at: www. flinders.edu.au/CDIP (accessed July 2005).

11 Wear D. Insurgent multiculturalism: rethinking how and why we teach culture in medical education. *Acad Med*. 2003; **78**: 549–54.

12 Kai J, Bridgwater R, Spencer J. 'Just think of TB and Asians', that's all I ever hear: medical learners' views about training to work in ethnically diverse society. *Med Educ*. 2001; **35**: 250–6.

13 Greenhalgh T, Helman C, Chowdhury M. Health beliefs and folk models of diabetes in British Bangaldeshis: a qualitative study. *BMJ*. 1998; **316**: 978–83.

14 Green AR, Betancourt JR, Carrillo JE. Integrating social factors into cross-cultural medical education. *Acad Med*. 2002; **77**: 193–7.

15 Irvine R, McPhee J, Kerridge IH. The challenge of cultural and ethical pluralism to medical practice. *MJA*. 2002; **176**: 174–5.

16 Joint Commission Resources. *Providing Culturally and Linguistically Competent Health Care*. Illinois: JCR; 2006.

17 Thomas L. Psychotherapy in the context of race and culture: an inter-cultural therapeutic approach. In: Fernanado S, editor. *Mental Health in a Multi-Ethnic Society*. Hove: Brunner-Routledge; 2002. pp. 172–90.

18 Henry B, Houston S, Mooney G. Institutional racism in Australian healthcare: a plea for decency. *Med J Aust*. 2004; **180**: 517–20.

19 Fernando S. *Mental Health, Race and Culture*. 2nd ed. Basingstoke: Palgrave; 2002.

20 Ferns P, Madden M. Training to promote race equality. In: Fernanado S, editor. *Mental Health in a Multi-Ethnic Society*. Hove: Brunner-Routledge; 2002. pp. 107–19.

21 University of Warwick Medical School. News. Available at: www2.warwick.ac.uk/fac/med/newsfront/?newsItem=094d43f0195291bb011952b3fa6705b1 (accessed April 2007).

22 The Transcult Psychiatry Unit, Curtin University, RACGP WA Research Unit. *Cultural Awareness Tool. Understanding Cultural Diversity in Mental Health*. 2002. Available at: www.mmha.org.au/mmha-products/books-and-resources/cultural-awareness-tool-cat/file (accessed January 2008).

23 Pilotto L, Duncan G, Anderson-Wurf J. Issues for clinicians training international medical graduates; a systemic review. *Med J Aust*. 2007; **187**: 225–8.

24 Association of Faculties of Medicine of Canada. *A Faculty Development Program for Teachers of International Medical Graduates*. 2006. Available at: www.afmc.ca/img/default_en.htm (accessed April 2008).

25 Chur-Hansen A. *Talking about Health and Illness: Australian slang*. 2006. Available at: www.adelaidetooutback.com.au/resources/pdf/adaptedcolloqbook2.pdf (accessed April 2008).

Index